Periodontics: A Synopsis

Periodontics:
A Synopsis

W.M.M. Jenkins BDS DDS FDSRCPS
Consultant in Periodontics
Glasgow Dental Hospital and School
Honorary Clinical Senior Lecturer
University of Glasgow

and

C.J. Allan BDS FDSRCPS MRD
Consultant in Restorative Dentistry
Dundee Dental Hospital and School
Honorary Senior Lecturer in Periodontology
University of Dundee

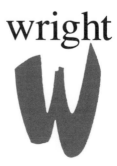

wright

OXFORD   AUCKLAND   BOSTON   JOHANNESBURG   MELBOURNE   NEW DELHI

Wright
An imprint of Butterworth-Heinemann
Linacre House, Jordan Hill, Oxford OX2 8DP
225 Wildwood Avenue, Woburn, MA 01801-2041
A division of Reed Educational and Professional Publishing Ltd

R   A member of the Reed Elsevier plc group

First published 1999
Reprinted 2000 (twice), 2001

© Reed Educational and Professional Publishing Ltd 1999

British Library Cataloguing in Publication Data
A catalogue record for this book is available from the British Library

Library of Congress Cataloguing in Publication Data
A catalogue record for this book is available from the Library of Congress

ISBN 0 7236 1062 2

For information on all Butterworth-Heinemann publications
please visit our website at www.bh.com

Composition by Scribe Design, Gillingham, Kent
Printed and bound by MPG Books Ltd, Bodmin, Cornwall

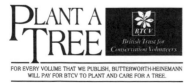

FOR EVERY VOLUME THAT WE PUBLISH, BUTTERWORTH-HEINEMANN
WILL PAY FOR BTCV TO PLANT AND CARE FOR A TREE.

Contents

Preface

The acquisition of knowledge in dentistry is perhaps more challenging today than ever before, while the requirement for continuing professional development has never been greater. There is, therefore, a growing need for texts which distil out essential concepts and make them accessible to the reader. This volume is an attempt to provide such a synopsis of current knowledge in the field of periodontics. It has been written primarily for the final year undergraduate to complement didactic teaching and clinical practice, but is also suitable for the practising clinician and the postgraduate needing to update basic knowledge or obtain a concise overview of clinical periodontology, prior to further study. We also hope that it will be read by dental hygienists who perform a pivotal role in the treatment of periodontal disease.

This text replaces our *Guide to Periodontics*, the third and last edition of which was published in 1994. Textbooks have a habit of expanding as each new edition succeeds the last – it is easy to add new information; more difficult, indeed sometimes painful to discard old material. *Guide to Periodontics* was no exception. Though never a large text, it was in danger of losing its focus through further revision. And so this new book, while incorporating much of the text and many of the illustrations of its predecessor, is entitled *A Synopsis* to reflect its concise format and the modern need for more incisive comment.

The biological basis and management of acute and chronic periodontal diseases are described within the wider context of dental care. A list of recommended further reading is provided near the end of the book, mostly comprising recent scientific reviews which expand the subject matter and serve as a starting point for readers who wish to explore the literature in greater depth.

We believe this description of current practice in periodontics and the concepts on which good clinical judgement is based will help the reader to develop a sound perspective on periodontal disease and its treatment.

W.M.M. Jenkins
C.J. Allan

Acknowledgements

Our sincere thanks and appreciation go to: Jeremy Bagg, Penny Hodge, Denis Kinane, Lone Sander and Robin Seymour for reading parts of the manuscript and for their helpful comments; and to staff in the Departments of Dental Illustration, Glasgow Dental Hospital and School and Medical Illustration, West Glasgow Hospitals University Trust for the clinical photographs and line drawings.

1

Structure and biology of the periodontium

The 'periodontium' comprises those structures which are directly involved in resisting forces applied to the teeth.

Tissues of the periodontium
- Gingiva
- Periodontal ligament
- Cementum
- Alveolar bone

The part of the periodontium which invests the coronal portion of the root is known as 'marginal periodontium'.

Gingiva

This is the fibrous mucosa surrounding the teeth and covering the coronal portion of the alveolar process (Figs 1.1 and 1.2). It is pink in colour in contrast to the deep red of alveolar mucosa. Gingiva is divisible into two parts: 'free' and 'attached'.

Free gingiva

This consists of the marginal part of the gingiva which can be deflected from the tooth surface by a probe inserted into the gingival sulcus. The apical boundary of the free gingiva is the free gingival groove, a shallow linear depression on the outer surface of the gingiva, parallel to the gingival margin, but found in only one-third of persons with normal gingiva.

Interdentally, the free gingiva extends to the contact point and forms the interdental papilla. Immediately below the contact point there is a slight depression, saddle or 'col'. The broader contact area of posterior teeth is associated with a larger col and separate buccal and lingual papillae may be recognized.

The epithelium of the free gingiva comprises three morphologically distinct compartments.

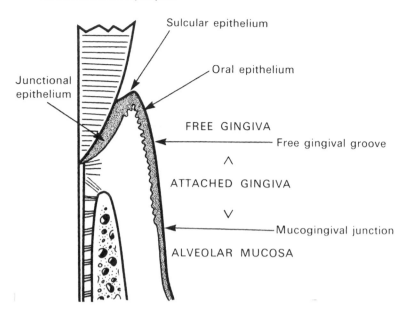

Fig. 1.1 Marginal periodontium.

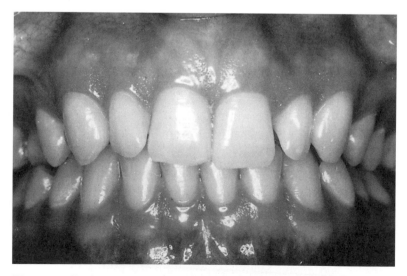

Fig. 1.2 Clinical appearance of normal gingiva: the gingiva has a 'knife-edge' margin; 'stippling' is apparent in some areas.

Epithelium of the free gingiva
- 'Oral gingival epithelium
- Oral sulcular epithelium
- Junctional epithelium

Oral gingival epithelium is continuous with and similar to the epithelium of attached gingiva. It extends up to the gingival margin but not into the sulcus. It has a stratified squamous morphology and keratinized surface. The underlying connective tissue forms papillary projections between which epithelial 'rete pegs' are found. These subsurface irregularities are responsible for the 'stippled' appearance of gingiva found in 40% of adults.

Oral sulcular (crevicular) epithelium is continuous with, and structurally similar to the oral epithelium of the gingiva, but is not keratinized. Below the contact point of adjacent teeth the sulcular epithelium is continuous with col epithelium, and resembles it closely. Sulcular and col epithelia are closely related to the tooth surface but are not attached to it. In health the gingival sulcus (crevice) is about 0.5 mm deep histologically.

Junctional epithelium is the epithelial collar which extends apically from the base of the sulcus to the amelocemental junction – a distance of about 2 mm. It is derived from reduced enamel epithelium and replenished by oral epithelium. It is a relatively thin layer of cells, tapering to its apical extremity, where it may be only one or two cells deep. The epithelial–connective tissue interface is smooth and rete pegs are absent. At the epithelial–tooth interface, an 'epithelial attachment' is formed, produced by cells of the junctional epithelium which coat the tooth surface with a basement membrane to which they attach by hemidesmosomes. Cell division in junctional epithelium is very rapid, the cells remaining immature as they migrate coronally from the basal layer, parallel to the tooth surface, to desquamate into the gingival sulcus (Fig. 1.3) a few days later. Keratinization does not take place.

The cells of the junctional epithelium are loosely knit, with wide intercellular spaces, and are much less adherent to one another than they are to the tooth surface. Junctional epithelium, therefore, is easily torn by insertion of a periodontal probe (Fig. 1.3).

An important feature of junctional epithelium is its permeability. This is a function not only of wide intercellular spaces but also of failure of the relatively undifferentiated cells to produce membrane coating granules which, in other types of epithelium, discharge their contents into the intercellular space to form an impermeable barrier.

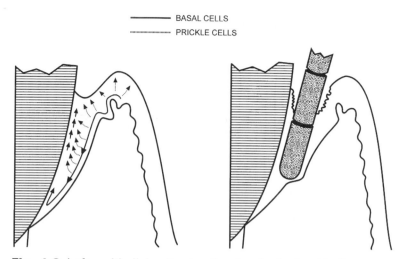

——————— BASAL CELLS

·············· PRICKLE CELLS

Fig. 1.3 Left: epithelial cell migration in gingival epithelium; the continuous line indicates how the basal layer of junctional epithelium is repopulated after wounding. Right: probing a healthy sulcus.

Epithelial differentiation. Although structurally different, the junctional, sulcular and oral epithelia are formed of cells which are fundamentally similar. These cells will adapt to their specific environment. The amount of contact which the epithelium makes with the tooth surface is one of the factors which determines how they will differentiate.

Probing a healthy sulcus. Although an inflammatory infiltrate is never completely absent, marginal gingiva is usually judged to be clinically healthy if it retains its normal pink colour, and if probing the sulcus fails to provoke bleeding. These conditions are described in this text as a 'physiological gingival sulcus'. The depth to which a normal healthy sulcus can be probed will depend on the diameter of the probe and the force applied, as well as tissue resistance. Beyond a depth of 0.5 mm the junctional epithelium will be torn (see Fig. 1.3), and discomfort may be felt when the probe tip approaches the connective tissue attachment at the amelocemental junction at a depth of 2–2.5 mm from the gingival margin. The normal range of probing depths is, therefore, 0.5–2.5 mm.

Attached gingiva

This extends from the apical border of the free gingiva to the mucogingival junction, which separates attached gingiva from

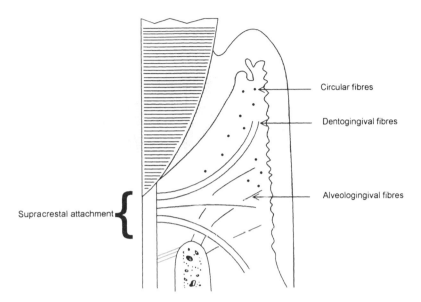

Fig. 1.4 Fibre types of the gingiva.

the alveolar mucosa. There is great variation in width of attached gingiva. It is usually widest (6.0 mm) on the lingual aspect of the first molar region of the mandible, and narrowest (0.5 mm) on the buccal aspect of the third molar region of the mandible. In the palate, there is no clear demarcation between the attached gingiva and palatal mucosa, both of which are keratinized structures. As attrition or loss of opposing teeth occurs, compensatory overeruption may take place, increasing the width of attached gingiva, the mucogingival junction being static while the gingival margin and alveolar bone maintain their relationship to the tooth by moving coronally with it.

Attached gingiva is bound by dense bundles of collagen fibres both to alveolar bone and, further coronally, to the root cementum. The attached gingival fibres, which are embedded in cementum, form part of the supracrestal fibre attachment (Fig. 1.4).

The supracrestal fibre attachment lies within the attached gingiva and is composed of fibres embedded in the narrow collar of cementum, normally about 1 mm wide, which extends from the amelocemental junction to the alveolar crest. From this portion of the root, 'dentogingival fibres' fan out into the free and attached gingiva, and 'transeptal fibres' run between teeth above the interdental septum (Fig. 1.5).

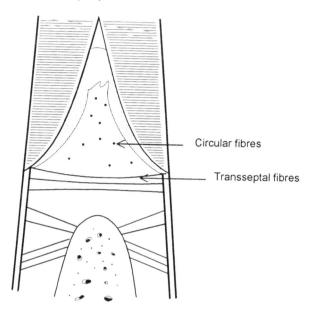

Circular fibres

Transseptal fibres

Fig. 1.5 Fibre types of the interdental gingiva.

In addition to these fibre bundles, circular fibres encircle the tooth within the free gingiva, and alveologingival fibres run in a coronal direction from the alveolar crest (see Fig. 1.4).

These various fibre bundles keep the gingiva tightly adapted to the tooth and alveolar process, and help to compensate for the inherent weakness of junctional epithelium.

Periodontal ligament

The periodontal ligament (membrane) attaches the tooth to alveolar bone. It is approximately 0.25 mm wide. Fibroblasts are the main cell type, but the main component is collagen, the principal fibres of which run in an apical direction from bone to root. The ends which are embedded in bone and cementum are known as Sharpey's fibres. Osteoblasts and cementoblasts may be present on the surfaces of bone and cementum respectively, and resorbing giant cells, derived from bone marrow, appear during phases of remodelling.

The main function of the periodontal ligament is to dissipate load and support the tooth during mastication. The ligament is a richly vascular and cellular tissue, metabolically very active and capable of considerable remodelling and repair. Increased function within physiological limits will cause a slight widening of the periodontal ligament, while reduced function has the opposite effect. Resistance to loading is achieved by hydro-dynamic damping (progressive displacement of blood from vessels), compression of periodontal ligament and deformation of alveolar bone, as well as stretching of the obliquely arranged principal collagen fibres which transmit stress to the bone as tension. Under vertically directed occlusal load, the entire periodontal ligament will be compressed and the maximum number of ligament fibres will be stretched. Lateral stress, on the other hand, causes a tipping movement around a fulcrum point approximately half-way between the alveolar crest and root apex: a relatively small number of periodontal fibres in the apical and cervical regions will become taut; the remaining ligament tissue may be unable to cushion the load adequately and pressure zones may be formed. Thus lateral stresses have a greater potential for injury to the periodontal structures.

Cementum

The entire root is covered in a layer of acellular cementum, about 0.05 mm thick, while only the apical third has a further coating of cellular cementum, which can be up to about 0.5 mm thick. At the amelocemental junction, cementum either abuts or overlaps the enamel, or occasionally stops slightly short of it, leaving some exposed dentine. Cementum is similar in compo-sition to bone but is avascular and not innervated.

Alveolar bone

Alveolar bone surrounds the roots of erupted teeth stopping about 1 mm short of the amelocemental junction. However, on buccal or lingual surfaces, if the tooth is outside the line of the arch, this distance may be considerably greater, forming a dehis-cence. In these circumstances, a longer supracrestal fibre attach-ment is present.

Defence mechanisms of the gingival sulcus

Gingival crevicular fluid (GCF) is an exudate, present in small amounts in health and in much larger quantities when inflammation is clinically apparent. GCF reaches the sulcus via the junctional epithelium, mixing with polymorphonuclear neutrophilic granulocytes (PMNs) and, to a lesser extent, monocytes which migrate by the same route as a result of chemotaxis from bacterial products.

The formation of bacterial plaque close to the gingival margin is a continuous process interrupted only briefly by oral hygiene procedures. The dentogingival junction represents a potential entry for toxic bacterial products reaching the underlying connective tissue. The following mechanisms help to maintain periodontal health.

Defence mechanisms
1. The anatomical epithelial seal preventing bacteria in the gingival sulcus from reaching the connective tissue.
2. Dynamic shedding of degenerated and infected junctional epithelial cells from the base of the sulcus.
3. Rapid repair of junctional epithelium following injury.
4. Flushing effect of gingival fluid.
5. The constant stream of PMNs, migrating through junctional epithelium into the gingival sulcus.
6. Antimicrobial substances within the GCF such as immunoglobulins and complement.

Pathogenesis

Definitions

Periodontal disease. This term, in its widest sense, includes all pathological conditions of the periodontium. It is, however, commonly used with reference to those inflammatory diseases which are plaque-induced and which affect the marginal periodontium: gingivitis and periodontitis.

Gingivitis is an inflammatory response of the gingiva without destruction of supporting tissues. The commonest form of gingival disease is chronic gingivitis, in which gingival enlargement and loss of resistance to probing occur. A gingival pocket may be present.

Periodontitis results from the apical extension of gingival inflammation to involve the supporting tissues. Destruction of the fibre attachment results in a periodontal pocket.

Development of chronic gingivitis
(Fig. 2.1(a) and (b))

There is no clear dividing line between gingival health and gingivitis, either in clinical or histopathological terms. Even gingiva that appears clinically healthy will show some evidence of vasculitis and perivascular collagen destruction. If plaque is allowed to accumulate, gingival fluid production will increase and polymorphonuclear neutrophil granulocytes will gather in large numbers in the junctional epithelium and gingival sulcus. After approximately 7 days of plaque accumulation, as the acute exudative response persists and collagen destruction continues, the connective tissues are infiltrated by T lymphocytes. After 10–21 days of continuous exposure to plaque, gingivitis becomes clinically evident (Fig. 2.1(a)): marginal erythema, a shallow gingival pocket or bleeding on probing are the first clinical signs. As gingivitis persists, plasma cells begin to accumulate within the infiltrated connective tissue. Chronic inflammatory cells may

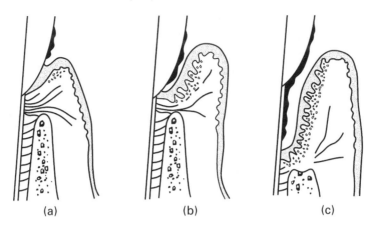

(a)   (b)   (c)

Fig. 2.1 The development of chronic gingivitis and periodontitis.
(a) Early gingivitis and supragingival plaque formation.
(b) Established chronic gingivitis with subgingival plaque in a
gingival pocket. (c) Chronic periodontitis with destruction of
periodontal ligament and alveolar bone and apical migration of
epithelial attachment.

overshadow the acute exudative response and, in due course, the
cellular infiltrate becomes dominated by plasma cells.

Gingivitis is initiated by supragingival plaque accumulation
(Fig. 2.1(a)) but, as gingival enlargement occurs, a subgingival
flora is created. With the apical advancement of subgingival
plaque, the junctional epithelium becomes detached from the
tooth surface to become pocket epithelium. The change from a
tooth-attached junctional epithelium to a non-adherent pocket
epithelium is accompanied by the formation and extension of
rete pegs into the infiltrated connective tissue (Fig. 2.1(b)).

Although collagen destruction always takes place within the
marginal gingiva adjacent to the tooth surface, in long-standing
gingivitis, fibroblast proliferation may occur outside the infiltrated zone, nearer the oral surface of the gingiva. This results
in fibrous gingival enlargement and masks the underlying
inflammation.

Clinical features of chronic gingivitis
(Fig. 2.2)

Marginal redness. The degree of erythema depends on the inten-
sity of the inflammatory response as well as the buccolingual thick-

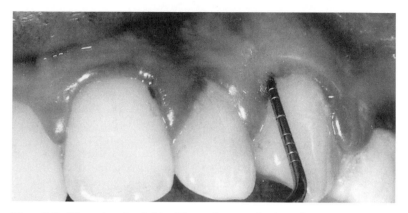

Fig. 2.2 Chronic gingivitis. There is marginal oedema, redness, loss of contour and bleeding on probing.

ness and consistency of gingival tissue. 'Thick' fibrotic gingival tissue will conceal the inflammation present on its inner surface.

Swelling. Blunting of interdental papillae and thickening of the free gingival margin is a result of oedema and/or a reactive increase in tissue cells (hyperplasia).

Bleeding on probing. This occurs when the friable pocket lining with its underlying dilated vasculature is traumatized. Bleeding on probing often precedes visual signs of inflammation such as redness or swelling.

Loss of stippling. This is a variable phenomenon, thought to be caused by the accumulation of oedema fluid.

Increased probing depth. The inflammatory reaction will result in gingival enlargement and/or loss of resistance to probing, both of which give rise to an increased probing depth beyond the norm of 0.5–2.5 mm.

Severity

Generally, in individuals with a normal host response to plaque, the severity of gingivitis simply reflects the level of plaque control. However, complex forms of gingivitis exist where the tissue response is exaggerated by an underlying local or systemic modifying factor and these individuals may exhibit a level of gingivitis not commensurate with the quantity of plaque. Some of these conditions have specific clinical or histopathological features which differentiate them from simple gingivitis (see Chapters 3 and 5).

The transition stage

Although gingivitis can develop quickly (within 10–21 days following withdrawal of plaque control measures), an equilibrium is usually established between the increased mass of bacteria and the host defences, maintaining a state of chronic gingivitis indefinitely. The transition from gingivitis to periodontitis may occur at any time, and may be gradual and imperceptible. It may be precipitated, either by a proportional increase in pathogenic organisms within the subgingival microflora, or impaired host resistance, or by both factors in combination. While it is thought that gingivitis is a necessary precursor to periodontitis, some individuals may develop periodontitis without gross evidence of marginal gingivitis.

In theory, destruction of supporting tissue should be recognized by probing, where the probe tip passes beyond the amelocemental junction to reach the base of the pocket. In practice, however, the amelocemental junction is often indistinct, and the base of the pocket 'soft' and ill-defined, so that choosing between a diagnosis of gingivitis or early periodontitis may be very difficult. The distinction is unlikely to be important to the clinician, since treatment is similar for both diagnoses.

Development of chronic periodontitis
(see Fig. 2.1(c))

Chronic periodontitis includes all the features of established gingivitis with a predominantly plasma cell infiltrate.

Inflammatory changes subjacent to the pocket epithelium and the residual junctional epithelium are accompanied by the destruction of gingival connective tissue, periodontal ligament and alveolar bone. The root surface is altered by loss of its outer cementoblast layer and shallow resorptive lesions of cementum may occur.

Destruction of the collagen fibre attachment apical to the junctional epithelium is followed by proliferation and apical migration of junctional epithelium on the root surface. Thus, a strand of junctional epithelium will always be present at the base of the pocket, denying bacteria access to the deeper connective tissues.

As subgingival plaque extends onto the root, the surface cementum may adsorb plaque endotoxins. These toxins may have an irritant effect on the overlying soft tissue, preventing repair, unless the surface layers of cementum are removed along with plaque and calculus deposits during treatment.

Clinical features of chronic periodontitis

(Figs 2.3, 2.4)

The formation of (pathological) pockets is common to both gingivitis and periodontitis. The distinguishing feature of

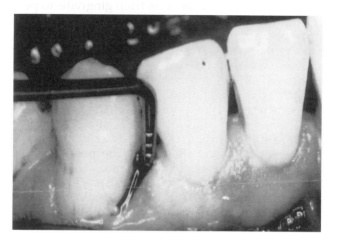

Fig. 2.3 Advanced chronic periodontitis in the absence of readily detectable gingival changes: the probe as an essential diagnostic tool.

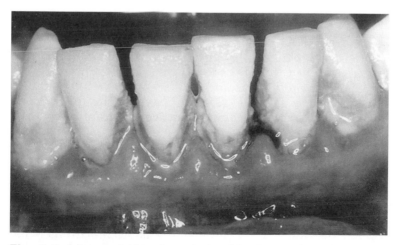

Fig. 2.4 Advanced chronic periodontitis. Gingival recession, tooth migration and mobility are present while marginal gingivitis persists owing to poor oral hygiene.

periodontitis is 'loss of connective tissue attachment'. In theory, this can be assessed clinically by measuring with a probe the distance between the amelocemental junction and the base of the pocket. Accurate measurement of attachment levels depends on the ability of the probe to 'split' the junctional epithelium and penetrate to the most coronally attached fibres. In practice, healthy gingival tissue will resist probing pressure and the probe tip may fail to reach the fibre attachment. Inflammation at the base of the pocket, on the other hand, may allow the probe tip to penetrate the connective tissue. Clinical attachment-level recordings are, thereby, subject to a significant measurement error, and this can be compounded by failure to locate the amelocemental junction accurately. The exact amount of attachment loss can be determined only by histology.

As attachment loss proceeds, and so long as gingival recession does not occur simultaneously at an equivalent rate, pockets will deepen. Nevertheless, some gingival recession frequently accompanies or follows destruction of the fibre attachment (Fig. 2.4) so that probing depths often fail to reflect the amount of attachment loss that has taken place.

Periodontitis is detected most readily with a probe, a blood-stained or purulent exudate being elicited by probing to the base of the pocket beyond the amelocemental junction (see Fig. 2.3).

Patterns of bone destruction

Bone destruction accompanies loss of fibre attachment and is essentially a *locally* destructive process, usually confined to a zone up to about 2 mm wide along the affected root surface (Fig. 2.5). Bone outside this zone lies beyond the effective radius of action of subgingival plaque. Thus, where the alveolar housing is thin, on buccal and lingual aspects and interdentally towards the necks of teeth, the apical extension of plaque will lead to destruction of the entire thickness of the alveolar process. This is so-called 'horizontal bone loss'. Frequently interdental bone, and less often buccal or lingual bone, is thicker than 2 mm so that resorption affects only the portion of bone lining the affected tooth surface with the formation of an 'angular' or 'vertical' bone defect. Thus the pattern of bone destruction within the mouth and around individual teeth reflects differences in bone morphology as well as the quantity and pathogenicity of plaque and its interaction with host defences.

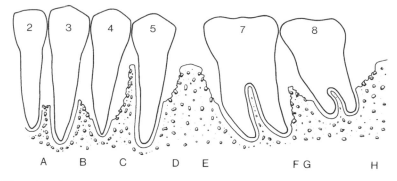

Fig. 2.5 Two-dimensional image of interdental bone defects A–H, which could originate as follows: A. the interdental septum is less than 2 mm wide: horizontal bone loss could arise from apical extension of plaque on one or both roots; B. bone loss on coronal half of 33 where interdental septum is less than 2 mm wide could be due to apical extension of plaque on 33 and 34 or 34 alone. Angular defect on mesial of 34 signifies more rapid disease progress on 34 than 33; C. broad interdental septum: mesial of 35 is not affected by periodontitis; D., E. very wide interdental bone allowing two separate angular defects; F., G. interdental septum broad enough apically to allow separate angular defects after narrower crestal bone totally destroyed; H. very wide bone defect. Resorbed surface outside radius of action of tooth-associated plaque, but could be caused either by subsequent mesial drift or bacterial invasion of pocket wall.

Suprabony pockets do not extend apical to the adjacent alveolar crest (see Fig. 2.1(c)). These pockets develop in association with horizontal bone loss, i.e. resorption of the entire thickness of the alveolar process.

Infrabony pockets extend apical to the adjacent alveolar crest. Infrabony (or 'intrabony') pockets are always associated with an angular bone defect and are usually classified according to the number of bone walls which surround the pocket. Figure 2.6 illustrates some of the many possible configurations. One of the commonest types of defect, the 'interdental crater' is illustrated separately in Figure 2.7 (the buccal and lingual walls form the sides of two two-walled pockets on adjacent proximal surfaces). This classification, while good in theory, is difficult to apply since most infrabony pockets taper towards the apex retaining additional 'bone walls' in the process (Fig. 2.6(e)). For treatment purposes, three-walled pockets show the greatest potential for bone-fill. At the opposite extreme a one-walled 'hemiseptum'

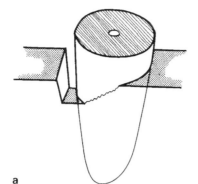
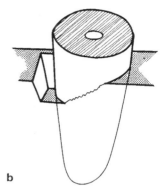
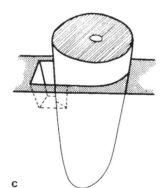
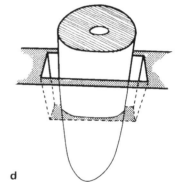
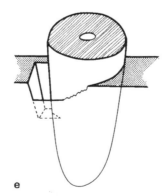

Fig. 2.6 Angular bone defects: (a) one proximal bone wall (hemiseptum), (b) two walls, (c) three walls, (d) four walls (funnel defect), (e) two walls coronally, three walls apically. (c) and (d) have good potential for bone-fill; (b) and (e) have rather less potential for bone-fill.

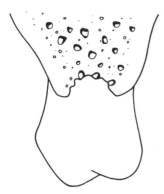

Fig. 2.7 Two-walled defect: interdental crater.

defect with a broad opening offers a poor framework for bone-fill, and attempts to eliminate the defect by bone resection would damage the support of the less affected adjacent tooth.

Complicating factors

Furcation lesions, periodontal–pulpal disease, gingival recession, tooth migration and hypermobility are all pathological features of advancing chronic periodontitis (see Fig. 2.4) and are dealt with in Chapters 13, 14, 17 and 18.

Terminal periodontitis

Untreated periodontitis may eventually give rise to acute painful episodes or culminate in exfoliation. The former may present as an acute periodontal abscess or as pulpitis due to toxic substances reaching the pulp from plaque deposits on the root surface. Pulp necrosis may also occur when apical vessels are affected by occlusal trauma in cases of advanced loss of support-ing tissue. Although such changes do not preclude attempts at treatment, they are usually indicative of deep-seated disease where extraction may be unavoidable.

Disease activity

Since all inflammatory processes, which have been investigated at the molecular level, are episodic with periods of destruction and repair interspersed, it is assumed that this pattern applies also to periodontitis. Thus, the expression 'periodontal disease activity' is used to describe the ongoing loss of connective tissue attachment which occurs during destructive phases. It would appear that most breakdown is characterized by destructive phases of small magnitude but high frequency, giving the appearance of continuous progression within a larger time frame, although large increments of destruction over short periods of time may also occur.

Predicting periodontal disease activity

Periodontal pockets, once formed, will persist indefinitely unless treated. On the other hand, progressive destruction is by no means inevitable and, at any point in time, a large proportion of diseased sites are inactive. This, of course, does not mean that signs of inflammation disappear during remission and reappear during periods of activity. Indeed, it must be stressed that bleeding from the base of the pocket on probing merely denotes the presence of inflammation and will occur in quiescent phases as well as during periods of progressive destruction.

Longitudinal studies have shown that, as one would expect, the risk of attachment loss at non-bleeding sites is low. When disease is already present, as revealed by bleeding on probing, the risk of progressive attachment loss is increased under certain circumstances.

Increased risk for progressive attachment loss at bleeding sites
1. General
   in older adults
   in smokers
   in various systemic disorders, e.g. diabetes
   in patients with existing widespread destruction
2. Localat
   at molar sites
   at proximal surfaces
   at angular bone defects
   at deep pockets
   at sites of severe attachment loss

Disease variability

Far from being well understood and highly predictable, gingivitis and periodontitis are diseases which exhibit enormous variability among those whom they afflict:

- Many sites and many individuals are very resistant to attachment loss, even when long-standing gingivitis is present.
- When attachment loss occurs, it may affect different sites in the same mouth to different extents. Thus, severe attachment loss, for example, may be generalized throughout the mouth, or may affect only a few sites.
- Rates of attachment loss can vary markedly between time periods, between individuals and between sites in one mouth.
- At some sites, even those affected by advanced destruction, attachment loss may appear to cease completely for an extended period of time.

3

Aetiology

Periodontal disease is initiated and maintained by bacterial plaque. The extent of tissue damage is dependent on the interaction between plaque bacteria and host defence mechanisms. Local environmental factors may favour the accumulation of bacterial plaque. Systemic or local modifying factors act by altering the host response to bacterial plaque.

The initiating factor – dental bacterial plaque

Plaque and gingivitis. The earliest deposit to form on a cleaned tooth surface is the acquired pellicle – a structureless film of salivary glycoproteins selectively adsorbed on to hydroxyapatite crystals. It forms within minutes on a tooth polished with pumice. The formation of pellicle is accompanied by bacterial colonization as microorganisms in saliva adsorb to the pellicle. After 3 or 4 hours, a thin layer of plaque, composed mainly of Gram-positive cocci (principally streptococci) will be established. These remain the predominant microorganisms for approximately 7 days, although, during this time, there is a proportional increase in Gram-positive rods and in Gram-negative cocci and rods, and, after 7 days, filaments, fusobacteria and spirilla are found in greater numbers. With further maturation, spirochaetes and vibrios appear, and if plaque accumulation continues uninterrupted for 10–21 days, frank gingivitis develops.

The microbiology of gingivitis. Generally, *Actinomyces* species and Gram-negative rods constitute a larger proportion of the microflora as gingivitis develops, but such is the variation from subject to subject and site to site that the specific presence of these organisms is not believed to be of aetiological significance. Gingivitis, therefore, is associated mainly with quantitative changes in bacterial plaque rather than overgrowth of specific microorganisms.

Plaque and periodontitis. Like gingivitis, periodontitis is caused by plaque, by subgingival down-growth of those bacteria best able to evade host defences and survive in a low-oxygen environment. The composition of subgingival plaque, therefore, differs from that of plaque on the adjacent visible tooth surfaces. For example, in subgingival plaque, Gram-positive bacteria are found in lower proportions and Gram-negative bacteria in higher proportions than in supragingival plaque. The subgingival flora comprises a layer of tooth-attached plaque as well as a loosely adherent component in direct association with the pocket epithelium. The tooth-attached plaque comprises mainly Gram-positive rods and cocci while the unattached plaque consists predominantly of Gram-negative organisms including motile forms. The relatively stagnant environment of the pocket will encourage the colonization of those bacteria not able to adhere readily to the tooth surface. Motile organisms, therefore, will be found in higher proportions within loosely adherent subgingival plaque than anywhere else in the mouth.

A subgingival flora, once established, is protected both from the natural cleansing action of tongue, lips, cheeks and saliva, and from toothbrushing. Yet, subgingival bacteria remain outwith the tissues where they control their own environment and can, to some extent, evade inflammatory and immune defence mechanisms.

The microbiology of periodontitis. There are over 300 bacterial species associated with the gingival sulcus and most of these organisms have been found in subgingival plaque. However, it is recognized that some subgingival bacteria will play a larger role than others. Those listed in Table 3.1 are common isolates, frequently constituting more than 2–3% and sometimes more than 50% of the cultivable subgingival flora, and possessing potent virulence factors. All, with the possible exceptions of *Actinobacillus actinomycetemcomitans* and *Porphyromonas gingivalis*, are members of the normal oral flora and are found, albeit in much smaller proportions, in healthy sites. Longitudinal cultural studies have sought to link a high proportional recovery of certain organisms with phases of progressive periodontitis. However, these studies suggest that disease activity is associated with different bacterial species in different patients. No one species has been shown to be present in all cases of any clinical category of periodontitis.

Microbial virulence factors. The mechanisms by which bacteria may provoke an inflammatory and immune response and cause tissue destruction are complex. Bacterial invasion of the tissues, if it occurs at all, is thought to be relatively unimportant. Instead, tissue damage is sustained mainly by penetration of the tissues by various soluble substances produced by plaque bacteria. These

Table 3.1 Common isolates from subgingival plaque (in alphabetical order)

Bacterium	Characteristics		
Actinobacillus actinomycetemcomitans	Gram –ve	Non-motile	Capnophilic* rod
Bacteroides forsythus	Gram –ve	Non-motile	Anaerobic rod
Campylobacter rectus	Gram –ve	Motile	Anaerobic curved rod
Eikenella corrodens	Gram –ve	Non-motile	Capnophilic* rod
Eubacterium species	Gram +ve	Non-motile	Anaerobic rod
Fusobacterium nucleatum	Gram –ve	Non-motile	Anaerobic rod
Peptostreptococcus micros	Gram +ve	Non-motile	Anaerobic coccus
Porphyromonas gingivalis	Gram –ve	Non-motile	Anaerobic rod
Prevotella intermedia	Gram –ve	Non-motile	Anaerobic rod
Selenomonas species	Gram –ve	Motile	Anaerobic curved rod
Treponema species	Gram –ve	Motile	Anaerobic spirochaete

* Capnophilic = CO_2 dependent

'toxins' have wide-ranging effects: in addition to toxic effects on host cells and enzymic degradation of tissue, chemotactic and antigenic effects occur, as well as activation or suppression of inflammatory and immune mechanisms, and stimulation of bone resorption.

Host defence mechanisms

Saliva

Saliva contains antimicrobial factors, such as lysozyme, and the constant production of saliva, in conjunction with swallowing, helps to prevent the build-up of supragingival plaque.

Epithelium

Sulcular, junctional and pocket epithelia form a barrier against ingress of bacteria, and epithelial cells produce mediators which initiate and maintain inflammatory and immune reactions.

The inflammatory response

The inflammatory response is vitally important to maintain the integrity of the periodontal tissue and prevent overwhelming infection. It comprises a vascular response, complement activation, emigration of polymorphonuclear neutrophil leucocytes (PMNs) and macrophages, and fibroblast activity.

The vascular response. Dilatation of post-capillary venules allows fluid exudate to dilute and expel bacterial products from the periodontal tissues and pocket, together with non-adherent plaque bacteria.

Complement activation. The complement system comprises a variety of proteins which circulate in an inactive form and are activated in an enzyme cascade to perform many different roles. A very important function of activated complement is opsonization of bacteria for phagocytosis. Although bacteria themselves, or their products, may be capable of activating complement, activation by antibody, already bound to these antigens, appears to be more efficient.

Emigration of PMNs. Most PMNs pass through the gingiva into the sulcus or pocket to kill bacteria by phagocytosis or secretion of toxic substances. PMNs have a major role in host defence against plaque bacteria.

Emigration of macrophages. Most macrophages remain in the tissues, where they phagocytose and kill bacteria, remove degraded tissue, and control the inflammatory reaction. Some macrophages are transported via the lymphatic system to present antigen to lymphocytes for induction of immune responses in the regional lymph nodes.

Fibroblast activity. Fibroblasts within the infiltrated zone produce collagenase to break down collagen and allow free movement of inflammatory cells. Fibroblasts peripheral to the infiltrated tissue produce collagen and ground substance to wall off the inflammatory reaction.

The immune response

On recognition of foreign antigens, lymphocytes are stimulated to reproduce, giving rise to a larger pool of cells which are programmed to protect the host by humoral or cell-mediated mechanisms.

The humoral response. Plaque bacteria and their products are antigenic and are transported by macrophages from the inflamed tissue to local lymph nodes. On recognition of foreign antigen, B lymphocytes are stimulated to reproduce, and ultimately differentiate into plasma cells which secrete antibody into the blood stream. Antibody can inactivate plaque products, opsonize bacteria for phagocytosis and fix (activate) complement at the bacterial surface. In severe periodontal disease, high levels of circulating antibody against several species of bacteria can be detected. Following treatment, antibody levels decline. Plasma cells are also found in the infiltrated zone, often in large numbers, produced locally by lymphocytes. These plasma cells also secrete antibody, but their role in the immune response is uncertain.

The cell-mediated response. Cell-mediated immunity involves T-lymphocyte activation principally against intracellular pathogens, fungi and tumour cells. This form of immune response may occur in periodontal disease, although its function is unclear. T lymphocytes may have a regulatory role in antibody production, T-helper lymphocytes stimulating B lymphocytes to become antibody-producing plasma cells, and T-suppressor lymphocytes having the opposite effect.

Mediators

The activities of the inflammatory and immune responses and of periodontal tissue cells are controlled and linked by a variety of soluble mediators which are synthesized and secreted by cells of all types involved in host defence. Prominent among these mediators are the cytokines which transmit information between cells.

Bystander damage

The destruction of periodontal tissue may be caused, as previously noted, by the direct toxic action of bacteria. It is likely, however, that some of the damage is caused by the defence mechanism itself. For example, some mediators induce fibroblasts to produce collagenase and osteoclasts to resorb bone, and the enzymes and toxins secreted by PMNs and macrophages are harmful to surrounding tissue. Host defence mechanisms, therefore, are both protective and destructive, although in most cases the tissue damage sustained is minor relative to the protection provided.

Progression of periodontitis

A normal, intact host response would appear to be compatible with, at worst, slowly progressive periodontal disease. However, fluctuations in the capacity of various components of the host response to deal with the bacterial challenge may alter the characteristics of periodontal disease. For example, abnormalities in PMN function have been associated with rapidly destructive disease.

Local environmental factors

Calculus. Mineralization within plaque results in calculus formation. Calcification may commence within 24 hours of plaque accumulation, but the rate of formation is very variable between individuals. Subgingival calculus forms more slowly and, being firmly attached, is usually more difficult to remove. Calculus is always covered by plaque and retains toxic bacterial products. The removal of calculus is, therefore, of fundamental importance in periodontal treatment.

Dental morphological factors. The palatal groove, occasionally present on upper incisors, may accumulate plaque and become the focus of a narrow destructive lesion of the periodontium. Likewise, following gingival recession, plaque may accumulate undisturbed in the mesial fossa of the upper first premolar, just apical to the contact point.

Soft-tissue factors. The presence of a fraenum, attached close to the gingival margin, may impede satisfactory plaque control, as may a shallow vestibule (see Chapter 17).

Crowding. Crowded, malpositioned teeth may present difficulties in plaque control, and access for scaling procedures may be restricted.

Restorations and prostheses. This will be described in greater detail in Chapter 21. Restorative materials, with the exception of glazed porcelain, accumulate plaque more rapidly than intact enamel. Unpolished or unglazed restorations will accumulate plaque more readily. Poor crown and pontic contour, especially excessive axial contours, favour plaque retention near the gingival margin. Above all, subgingival restorations, especially those with defective or overhanging margins, may have a profound effect on periodontal health by retaining plaque within a gingival pocket. Partial-denture wearers will accumulate more plaque on their remaining teeth because of impaired natural cleansing.

Systemic modifying factors

A number of systemic conditions have been shown to increase the severity of plaque-induced periodontal diseases. Examples are listed below.

Pregnancy

It is well established that there is an increase in severity of gingivitis during pregnancy until the eighth month, when the severity of gingivitis begins to decline. The gingival changes appear to be caused by the effect of increased levels of oestrogen and progesterone on the microvasculature and immune system. Apart from generalized gingival changes, a pregnancy granuloma may occur (Fig. 3.1). This hyperplastic lesion has the same histology as the 'pyogenic granuloma'. Newly formed capillaries dominate the lesion.

Puberty

The severity and extent of gingivitis tend to increase in childhood and reach a peak at puberty, before declining during adolescence. Hormonal changes are considered to be partly responsible for this occurrence. The peak at this age group may also be attributed to the end of the mixed dentition stage and the positive effect of improving social awareness on plaque control.

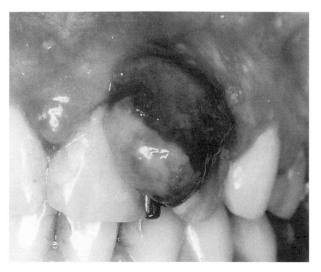

Fig. 3.1 Ulcerated pregnancy epulis. This lesion reveals the concurrence of the initiating factor (plaque) with a local environmental factor (overhanging cervical margin of the gold inlay in 21) and a systemic modifying factor (pregnancy).

Diabetes mellitus

Diabetes is associated with a variety of defects in host defence: degeneration of gingival blood vessel walls, altered collagen metabolism, and deficient chemotactic, phagocytic and bactericidal activity of PMNs. Thus, diabetes carries an increased risk of severe gingivitis and periodontitis. This applies both to insulin-dependent and non-insulin-dependent forms of the disease. The relationship between diabetes and periodontal disease is more likely to be observed if diabetic control is poor.

Blood dyscrasias

Agranulocytosis and neutropenia. Agranulocytosis and neutropenia, including cyclic neutropenia, are associated with an increased severity of gingivitis, necrotic ulceration and advanced periodontal destruction.

Acute leukaemia. Gingival enlargement, ulceration, inflammation, purpura and severe bleeding are characteristic of some cases of acute leukaemia attributable to the infiltration of malignant cells, neutropenia, impaired phagocytosis, platelet deficiency and decreased effectiveness of immune mechanisms.

If the patient survives long enough, advanced periodontal destruction may also be noted. Cytotoxic drugs and antibiotics may have a variety of adverse or beneficial effects on the clinical periodontal picture.

Human immunodeficiency virus (HIV)

HIV-seropositive individuals appear to be vulnerable to a chronic persistent erythematous gingivitis, acute necrotizing ulcerative gingivitis (ANUG) and an aggressive necrotizing periodontitis. These conditions are described more fully in Chapter 20.

Hereditary and genetic factors

In common with many other diseases, susceptibility to periodontal disease in the general population may, to some extent, be genetically determined. Evidence in favour of a genetic predisposition is strongest for localized juvenile periodontitis. There are, in addition, a number of recognized congenital diseases with periodontal manifestations.

Hereditary gingival fibromatosis is a rare condition, possibly transmitted by a dominant gene, where there is gross fibrous enlargement of the gingivae in response to plaque accumulation. Affected individuals are usually otherwise healthy.

Down's syndrome may be associated with greater severity of gingivitis and periodontitis, in both the deciduous and permanent dentition, perhaps due to altered connective tissue metabolism, or functional defects of PMNs and macrophages.

Hyperkeratosis palmaris et plantaris (Papillon–Lefèvre syndrome), hypophosphatasia, leucocyte adhesion deficiency and Chédiak–Higashi syndrome are examples of rare conditions, inherited as autosomal recessive traits, which are associated with rapidly destructive plaque-induced periodontal disease in both the deciduous and permanent dentition. In some of these conditions the pathogenic mechanism is well understood. For example, in leucocyte adhesion deficiency, PMNs cannot adhere to capillary endothelium, and thus cannot enter the tissues.

Drug ingestion

Oral contraceptive drugs have been shown to cause an increased severity of gingivitis and, after prolonged use, greater loss of attachment.

Three drugs are frequently associated with fibrous gingival overgrowth: the anti-epileptic drug phenytoin, the immunosuppressant drug cyclosporin, which is used primarily in organ transplantation, and the calcium channel blocker nifedipine, which is a peripheral and coronary vasodilator, used in the treatment of angina pectoris and hypertension.

There is a wide range of individual patient response to these drugs, to some extent explained by dosage and oral hygiene levels. Gingival overgrowth has been reported in up to 65% of patients taking phenytoin, up to 85% taking cyclosporin and up to 45% taking nifedipine. It is well established that other calcium channel blockers may cause gingival overgrowth, although less commonly than nifedipine.

All drugs which cause fibrous gingival overgrowth appear to inhibit the cellular uptake of calcium, causing a reduction in collagenase activity. Gingival enlargement, therefore, results from the accumulation of increased extracellular matrix, mainly collagen.

Treatment measures include oral hygiene instruction, professional cleaning, withdrawal or substitution of the drug and, if necessary, surgical excision.

Smoking

Cigarette smoking is positively associated with ANUG and with an increased prevalence and severity of periodontitis. This may be partly attributable to poorer oral hygiene among smokers compared to non-smokers. However, smoking *per se* is now known to be a major risk factor for periodontitis because of the systemic effects of smoking on host defence mechanisms. These effects include peripheral vasoconstriction, inhibition of PMN chemotaxis and phagocytosis, reduced antibody production, decreased T-helper/suppressor cell ratio and diminished fibroblast activity. Any of these mechanisms could be responsible for the predisposition of smokers to ANUG (see Chapter 20) and the increased prevalence and severity of periodontitis compared with non-smokers. Smoking has also been shown to inhibit healing after treatment. These harmful effects of smoking appear to be linked both to the duration of the habit and the amount smoked, while periodontal health in former smokers is intermediate between that of smokers and non-smokers.

Although smokers are predisposed to ANUG and periodontitis, they seem to be more resistant than non-smokers to chronic gingivitis, and exhibit less gingival bleeding on probing. This may be less of a paradox than it seems: in the presence of plaque, failure to maintain an effective inflammatory response, manifest as chronic gingivitis, could promote eventual gingival necrosis or breakdown of the underlying supporting tissues.

Local modifying factors

Lip morphology and mouthbreathing

Lip-apart posture, with reduced coverage of the upper incisor segment, often results in marked erythema of the free and attached gingivae on both labial and palatal aspects. Mouthbreathing causes similar gingival changes, but only on palatal gingivae. While this cause and effect relationship is beyond dispute, the mechanism for these changes is not fully understood. Certainly, the upper anterior teeth will not be fully exposed to salivary antimicrobial agents, and this, together with lack of functional cleansing, may result in increased plaque accumulation and, thereby, increased gingivitis. According to this theory, the lip posture or mouthbreathing habit acts as a local environmental factor enhancing plaque accumulation. Alternatively, dry gingivae may be more susceptible to the presence of plaque. Indeed, drying of the gingivae is likely to result in inflammatory changes, even when no plaque is present.

Inflammatory gingival enlargement is common in cases of inadequate lip coverage, and may, perhaps, be attributed to the absence of normal lip pressure.

Periodontal trauma

Any excessive force causing sufficient tooth displacement will produce a traumatic lesion of the supporting structures. Orthodontic forces and occlusal stress are the commonest causes of periodontal trauma. Lesions with similar pathological features will be produced by all forms of periodontal trauma. The effect of adverse occlusal forces on the periodontium is described in the next chapter, including the possible role of occlusal trauma as a modifying factor in the pathogenesis of periodontal disease.

4

Trauma from occlusion

Trauma from occlusion (occlusal trauma) is an injury to any part of the masticatory system resulting from abnormal occlusal contact. In the periodontal context, occlusal trauma may take two forms:

1. Surface injury caused by deep overbite or food impaction (see Chapter 18).
2. Injury within the connective tissue attachment apparatus as a result of excessive occlusal force transmitted by the tooth to its supporting structures. It is this form of occlusal trauma which is discussed here.

Adaptive physiological response to occlusal force

When a tooth in traumatic occlusion is subjected repeatedly to excessive occlusal force, it moves within its periodontium in such a way that pressure and tension zones are created in the periodontal ligament. Reorganization within and adjacent to these zones will lead either to an increase in tooth mobility or to progressive repositioning (migration) of the tooth in the direction of the applied force, or both, until the effect of the force is nullified. If the tooth movement results in a bony dehiscence, gingival recession may follow (see Chapter 17). Whether the tooth becomes mobile or migrates away from the stress, will depend not only on the direction and duration of occlusal forces but also, to a large extent, on the support provided by tongue, lips and cheeks. In the incisor region, for example, although there is potential for teeth to drift forward under occlusal stress or due to tongue pressure, reciprocal pressure from the lips helps to maintain these teeth in a stable position within the so-called neutral zone. If an anterior tooth is traumatized by the occlusion when lip support is good, it will be 'jiggled' between

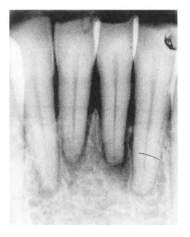

Fig. 4.1 Traumatic periodontal lesions and chronic periodontitis in a bruxist patient. Radiograph of the lower incisors reveals: a reduction in bone height due to inflammatory periodontal disease; widened periodontal ligament spaces due to occlusal stress; absence of lamina dura around the apices, indicative of ongoing trauma.

the opposing teeth and lips, and become mobile. If lip support is poor, however, the tooth may migrate forwards or procline.

The mechanism for developing tooth mobility following the application of an excessive force involves an increase in periodontal ligament width, and bone resorption with loss of definition of lamina dura. These features may be observed on radiographs only if the X-ray beam has transected the affected zones of the periodontium (Fig. 4.1). Adaptation is complete when the magnitude of tooth mobility or the extent of tooth migration is sufficient to accommodate or annul the displacing force. Migrated teeth will stabilize in their new position. Teeth which have maintained their positions in the arch and have accommodated to the force by increasing tooth mobility will remain mobile. When adaptation is complete, new lamina dura of both migrated and hypermobile teeth may be observed radiographically, but the increased periodontal ligament space of hypermobile teeth will persist.

The development of tooth mobility or migration may, in theory, occur entirely as a physiological process if the displacing force is introduced gently, but often these tooth movements represent 'recovery phenomena' following one or more episodes of occlusal trauma.

Diagnosis of occlusal trauma

The clinical diagnosis of occlusal trauma should be reserved for symptoms of periodontal pain or discomfort where the history and clinical examination support an occlusal aetiology. Periodontal occlusal trauma is an injury not unlike a traumatic injury to any other part of the body, and is characterized by a zone of increased vascularity, vascular permeability, haemorrhage and thrombosis; in severe cases, also by hyalinization of periodontal ligament with undermining resorption of bone and cementum; and, in extreme cases, by necrosis and abscess formation.

Occlusal trauma is occasionally caused solely by increased functional demands – by the onset of bruxism, for example, or by a new restoration creating a premature contact. More commonly, however, trauma results from a reduction in periodontal support and subsequent failure to withstand normal or increased occlusal stresses.

Occlusal trauma is often transient and quickly followed by the adaptive responses outlined above, so that treatment may never be sought. This is probably a common sequence of events following the introduction of an inadequately contoured restoration. Except where pain is present, therefore, occlusal trauma is a diagnosis which must often be made in retrospect on the basis of tooth mobility or migration and the radiographic appearance of a widened periodontal ligament (see Fig. 4.1), together with evidence of occlusal disharmony to support an occlusal aetiology. In this situation, the increased tooth mobility and widened periodontal ligament space are the clinical and radiographic manifestations, respectively, of an adaptive response by the periodontium to accommodate the excessive forces acting on the tooth. By this time, there is probably no longer an actual traumatic lesion present, but rather a periodontal ligament which is functionally orientated to accommodate the excessive forces.

Occasionally, however, trauma may not be self-limiting: *increasing* mobility, persistent discomfort or tenderness, and radiographic signs, such as absence of lamina dura or progressive root resorption, point to a diagnosis of persistent occlusal trauma.

Occlusal trauma as a modifying factor

The potential for occlusal trauma to initiate or exacerbate inflammatory periodontal disease was the subject of much speculation until a series of investigations was conducted in squirrel monkeys and beagle dogs in the 1970s. A limited number of well-controlled human studies have also been performed.

Findings from these animal and human studies are summarized as follows:

1. Occlusal trauma may result in widening of the periodontal ligament, loss of crestal bone and tooth mobility, all without loss of attachment, and all of which are reversible when the tooth is relieved of stress.
2. Occlusal trauma *does not* initiate or exacerbate gingivitis.
3. Occlusal trauma *does not* initiate chronic periodontitis or convert gingivitis to periodontitis.
4. Occlusal trauma *does not* initiate further loss of connective tissue attachment in a tooth with a reduced but healthy periodontium.
5. Occlusal trauma in combination with chronic marginal periodontitis results in greater tooth mobility and alveolar bone loss (but not necessarily more loss of connective tissue attachment) than either trauma or inflammation alone.
6. Bone loss and mobility due to trauma may be reversible, but only once inflammation has been controlled, since persistent inflammation may inhibit crestal bone regeneration.

What these studies have failed to do is to determine whether occlusal trauma in combination with chronic periodontitis may result in greater loss of connective tissue attachment. On that issue, the experimental work was inconclusive. There is, furthermore, no satisfactory evidence that occlusal therapy can improve the prognosis for inflammatory periodontal disease.

Where progressive occlusal trauma exists, it should be treated to relieve pain or discomfort and to control increasing tooth mobility or migration. Occlusal therapy is discussed in Chapter 18.

5

Classification and epidemiology

A classification provides a useful framework to view the spectrum of disorders which may be included in the term 'periodontal disease'. No classification, however, has yet been devised which has achieved wide acceptance. The one illustrated in Table 5.1 includes a wide range of established and proposed clinical entities some of which are considered in more detail in the text below.

Plaque-associated diseases

'Plaque-associated diseases' are those inflammatory conditions of the periodontium with bacterial plaque as the primary aetiological agent.

Simple gingivitis is the common form of chronic gingivitis where no identifiable modifying factors are present.

Complex gingivitis occurs when specific local or systemic modifying factors exist. These are listed in Table 5.1 and described in Chapter 3.

Reactive epulides are localized polypoidal gingival lesions which originate from inflamed gingiva, often from the supracrestal fibre attachment and, therefore, from beyond the base of the gingival or periodontal pocket. They are assumed to result from the stimulating effect of dental plaque on a localized area of particularly sensitive connective tissue. Epulides may be sessile or pedunculated and can be classified as: (1) the pyogenic granuloma (see Fig. 3.1), which is characterized by extensive endothelial and fibroblastic proliferation associated with a dense chronic inflammatory infiltrate; (2) the fibrous epulis, consisting of dense fibrous tissue, occurring either *de novo* or due to maturation of a pyogenic granuloma; or (3) the giant cell epulis, resembling a pyogenic granuloma clinically and histologically with the addition of large numbers of multinucleated giant cells. The reactive epulides are treated usually by local excision, as described in Chapter 11.

Table 5.1 *Classification of periodontal diseases*

Plaque-associated diseases
Gingivitis
  Chronic
    Simple gingivitis
    Complex gingivitis
    e.g. mouthbreathing gingivitis
      pregnancy gingivitis
      puberty gingivitis
      leukaemic gingivitis
      drug-induced gingival hyperplasia
      hereditary gingival fibromatosis
    Reactive epulides
  Acute
    Necrotizing ulcerative gingivitis

Periodontitis
  Chronic
    Adult periodontitis
    Early onset periodontitis
      prepubertal periodontitis
        localized
        generalized
      juvenile periodontitis
        localized
        generalized
    Refractory periodontitis
  Acute
    Necrotizing ulcerative periodontitis
    Periodontal abscess

Non-plaque-associated diseases
Traumatic
  Occlusal trauma
  Gingival recession
Infective
  Acute herpetic stomatitis
Immunological
  Desquamative gingivitis

Acute necrotizing ulcerative gingivitis is a destructive form of gingivitis characterized by necrotic ulceration of the papillary, marginal and, occasionally, attached gingivae. It is described fully in Chapter 20.

Periodontitis is thought to comprise a family of related but distinct diseases that differ in precise aetiology, natural history and response to therapy. Whereas different forms of gingivitis are differentiated according to the influence of modifying factors, periodontitis is classified, less convincingly, mainly by age of onset and severity, since its precise aetiology is insufficiently understood. Nevertheless, periodontal literature is replete with references to different types of periodontitis. Perhaps the best that can be said of classifications of periodontitis is that, by providing a range of case definitions, they facilitate communication.

Adult periodontitis is the commonest form of periodontitis. It is considered to have its onset during or after adolescence, to progress relatively slowly compared to early-onset forms, and is unlikely to become clinically significant until the mid-thirties. However, the rate of attachment loss may increase at any time. In cross-sectional surveys of the general population, adult periodontitis is responsible for the majority of cases identified with advanced destructive disease. Adult periodontitis has not been linked to impaired host defence mechanisms.

Early-onset periodontitis (see Chapter 15) comprises those forms of the disease which are characterized by advanced destruction in childhood, adolescence or early adulthood. Advanced destruction in prepubertal children has been described as 'prepubertal periodontitis' and in adolescents or young adults as 'juvenile periodontitis'. Early-onset types of periodontitis have been linked to specific subgingival microfloras, to impairment of immune and inflammatory mechanisms, and to familial distributions. These associations are strongest for localized juvenile periodontitis.

Refractory periodontitis is a term which may be applied to any form of chronic periodontitis, early-onset or adult, which is either unresponsive to treatment or rapidly recurrent in spite of apparently appropriate therapy and good plaque control.

On the whole, with the exception of localized juvenile periodontitis, the various forms of chronic periodontitis are poorly characterized. There is considerable overlap and a precise diagnosis is frequently impossible: the time lapse between onset and diagnosis may be unknown; different diagnoses may be appropriate for different teeth in one mouth; and the influence of concurrent systemic disease may be difficult to assess. Indeed, periodontitis may also be conceived as a single disease with an infinite range of manifestations existing along a continuum; and attempts to split this disease into too many separate parts may create subdivisions without a biological basis. In any case, failure to make a definitive diagnosis should not prove to be a barrier to therapy, since all forms of chronic periodontitis share a common approach to treatment.

Necrotizing ulcerative periodontitis is a term of fairly recent origin, used to describe a situation where periodontitis and acute necrotizing ulcerative gingivitis (ANUG) coexist, in some cases because recurrent ANUG has apparently progressed to periodontitis. In the later stages of HIV infection, when the patient's immune system is severely compromised, gingival ulceration with necrosis of underlying soft tissue and alveolar bone may lead to advanced gingival recession and tooth exfoliation. Pain and spontaneous bleeding are common. This condition is sometimes described as HIV-associated periodontitis (see Chapter 20).

Periodontal abscesses are acute suppurative inflammatory lesions associated with destruction of the attachment apparatus (see Chapter 20).

Non-plaque-associated diseases

Non-plaque-associated diseases may occur independently or concurrently with plaque-associated disease. They include traumatic lesions, infections and immunological conditions, as listed in Table 5.1, as well as pathological processes which may affect the periodontal tissue but are not usually considered to be forms of periodontal disease; for example, cysts, neoplasms, renal osteodystrophy, hyperparathyroidism and contact sensitivity reactions. For an extensive review of non-plaque-associated diseases affecting the periodontium, the reader is referred to Newman *et al.* (1993).

Epidemiology

Epidemiological studies are carried out to determine population trends in the occurrence and distribution of periodontal disease. When large populations are compared, differences in gingivitis levels may be revealed which are largely attributable to differences in oral hygiene. Differences in levels of periodontitis between populations, however, are usually much less pronounced, reflecting the important role of host response factors which are often present in equal measure in different populations.

Prevalence and severity

The term 'prevalence' should serve to indicate, for a given age group, the proportion of the population affected by a given degree of severity of periodontal disease.

Gingivitis. Gingivitis is common in children, and was found in 36% of 3 year olds, 64% of 5 year olds, 97% of 10 year olds and 74% of 15 year olds in Sweden (Hugoson et al., 1981). The high prevalence in 10 year olds may be attributable to deterioration in the gingival condition of exfoliating teeth, and the lowered prevalence at 15 years to the effect of increased social awareness on oral hygiene. There is a further rise in gingivitis prevalence in adulthood.

Periodontitis. Sjödin and Matsson (1994), in a radiographic analysis of 2017 9-year-old Swedish children, found that 4.5% had evidence of marginal bone loss (distance between ameloce-mental junction and alveolar crest $\geq$ 2.5 mm) affecting their deciduous molars and canines.

In teenage populations, there is wide agreement that large amounts of periodontal destruction are unusual, but minor amounts may be quite common. In a 5-year longitudinal study of 167 British adolescents, initially 14 years of age, from a low socio-economic area, Clerehugh et al. (1990) determined the prevalence of attachment loss by examining the mesial surfaces of first molars, first premolars and central incisors for evidence of a reduction in attachment level of 1 mm or more. The prevalence of attachment loss was calculated at three time points:

Prevalence of attachment loss $\geq$ 1 mm

	Subject prevalence	Site prevalence
14 years	3%	< 1%
16 years	37%	7%
19 years	77%	31%

Attachment loss amounting to 2 mm affected only 3% of the group at 16 years and 14% at 19 years.

The data for 552 dentate adult subjects, illustrated in Table 5.2, are from an epidemiological survey in 1993 of 584 randomly selected individuals, evenly distributed into age levels, from a medium sized town in Sweden (Hugoson et al., 1998). Following a detailed clinical and radiographical examination, these individuals were assigned to one of five periodontal disease groups, the inclusion criteria for which are summarized below:

Group 1 – negligible signs of inflammation and no proximal surface bone loss.

Group 2 – generalized gingivitis but essentially no proximal surface bone loss.

Group 3 – generalized early bone loss (less than one-third of normal bone height).

Group 4 – generalized moderate bone loss (one-third to two-thirds of normal bone height).

Group 5 – generalized advanced bone loss (more than two-thirds of normal bone height).

Table 5.2 *Number of dentate individuals of each age and the percentage distribution according to severity of periodontal disease (After Hugoson et al., 1998)*

Age (years)	Number of dentates	Percentages Periodontal disease groups				
		1	2	3	4	5
20	100	37	63			
30	102	39	58	3		
40	93	23	44	28	3	2
50	97	10	28	40	14	7
60	83	15	17	44	18	6
70	77	4	8	55	26	7
	552	22	38	27	10	3

Table 5.2 shows that, out of the entire sample, 22% were essentially free of periodontal disease (group 1), while a further 38% had gingivitis without significant evidence of bone loss (group 2). Generalized early marginal bone loss (group 3), affected 27%, while only 10% and 3% of the entire sample suffered from generalized moderate (group 4) and advanced bone loss (group 5), respectively. The prevalence and severity of bone loss increased with increasing age. Generalized early bone loss affected only 3% of 30 year olds, perhaps reflecting the prevalence of so-called generalized early-onset periodontitis (see Chapter 15). Generalized moderate bone loss was common only at older age levels affecting 14%, 18% and 26% of 50, 60, and 70 year olds. Generalized advanced bone loss was not diagnosed before age 40 years and was uncommon at all ages thereafter.

In extrapolating the results of this Swedish study to other parts of the world, it must be remembered that these data were collected from a population with a high level of dental awareness. Nevertheless, there is good agreement with cross-sectional studies of various other adult populations that *generalized* moderate or advanced bone loss is confined to 10–15% of the population.

The grouping of patients into one of 5 categories, above, according to their 'whole mouth scores', results in considerable smoothing of data and disguises the prevalence of different threshold levels of disease, i.e. the proportion of patients with at least one tooth surface affected beyond certain disease thresholds. For example, in this study, only 5% of 40 year olds had *generalized* bone loss exceeding one-third of average root length. However, in a different study, also of Swedish subjects, Papapanou *et al.* (1988) demonstrated that 38% of 35 year olds and 63% of 45 year olds had bone loss exceeding one-third of average root length (>5 mm bone level reduction), affecting at least one tooth surface.

References

Clerehugh, V., Lennon, M.A. and Worthington, H.V. (1990). 5-year results of a longitudinal study of early periodontitis in 14 to 19-year-old adolescents. *Journal of Clinical Periodontology*, **17**, 702–708.

Hugoson, A., Koch, G. and Rylander, H. (1981). Prevalence and distribution of gingivitis–periodontitis in children and adolescents. *Swedish Dental Journal*, **5**, 91–103.

Hugoson, A., Norderyd, O., Slotte, C. and Thorstensen, H. (1998). Distribution of periodontal disease in a Swedish adult population 1973, 1983 and 1993. *Journal of Clinical Periodontology*, **25**, 542–548.

Newman, H.N., Rees, T.D. and Kinane, D.F. (eds) (1993). *Diseases of the Periodontium*. Northwood: Science Reviews Limited.

Papapanou, P.N., Wennström, J.L. and Grondahl, K. (1988). Periodontal status in relation to age and tooth type. A cross-sectional radiographic study. *Journal of Clinical Periodontology*, **15**, 469–478.

Sjödin, B. and Matsson, L. (1994). Marginal bone loss in the primary dentition. A survey of 7–9-year-old children in Sweden. *Journal of Clinical Periodontology*, **21**, 313–319.

History, examination, diagnosis and prognosis

The purpose of history taking and examination is to arrive at a diagnosis and preliminary assessment of prognosis upon which a treatment plan may be based. The purpose of this chapter is to highlight specific elements in this process, the prognostic significance of which is frequently overlooked or misunderstood.

History

The clinician should concentrate initially on the main concerns of the patient and/or referring clinician. However, patients should also be questioned specifically about each of the common signs or symptoms of plaque-induced periodontal disease.

Signs and symptoms
- Gingival bleeding, pain, swelling and recession.
- Tooth mobility and migration.
- Bad breath and taste.

Bleeding

Gingival bleeding may occur spontaneously or during mastication or tooth cleaning. A sudden onset or deterioration, which might suggest an underlying systemic factor, should be noted.

Pain

Pain is a common presenting feature of periodontal abscesses and acute necrotizing ulcerative gingivitis, but an infrequent symptom of chronic periodontal disease. Thus, before attributing pain symptoms to a chronic periodontal condition, alternative explanations must be sought. These include acute periodontal lesions, caries, pulp and periapical disease, dentine hypersensitivity, and occlusal trauma.

Tooth mobility

Patients are not always aware of increased tooth mobility. It is commonly associated with one or more of the following:

Causes of tooth mobility
1. Marginal or apical inflammation.
2. Loss of connective tissue attachment and supporting bone, usually due to marginal periodontal disease but occasionally due to periapical disease.
3. Apical root resorption.
4. Increase in width of periodontal ligament, usually due to occlusal forces.

Patients who complain of, or are aware of mobility should be asked about its duration and whether it appears to have increased since first noted. Any masticatory difficulty due to mobility such as discomfort or food impaction should also be noted.

While mobility may be a sign of disease, it may also be a sign of physiological adaptation to reduced support or increased function, and should by no means be invariably interpreted as a sign of poor prognosis or indication for extraction. Patients may need to be reassured about this. However, *increasing* mobility may indicate rapid loss of support and a poor prognosis.

Some decrease in mobility may follow control of inflammation, occlusal adjustment and periodontal surgery (after a temporary increase in mobility). Although splinting may lead to some decrease in mobility, following removal of the splint, mobility will return gradually to previous levels. Decrease in mobility may be taken as a favourable prognostic indicator. However, when periodontal support is reduced, some mobility must be expected to persist in spite of thorough treatment including occlusal adjustment. If tooth mobility interferes with comfort or function, or seems to be increasing, splinting may be indicated.

Tooth migration

Patients are usually aware of migration of anterior teeth because of the development of spaces. Migration may take place even when the periodontium is healthy, although it is more likely when there has been loss of support. It reflects the disruption of the normal balance of forces acting on teeth (see Chapter 4). Migration may, therefore, be due to loss of an adjacent tooth, to functional or parafunctional occlusal stress, or activity of the oral musculature. It may occur without significant mobility. If orthodontic correction is possible, permanent retention will usually be required.

Medical history

A careful medical history must be taken from all patients and periodically updated. The principal objectives are:

Objectives of the medical history
1. To identify systemic factors which may help to account for the periodontal condition, i.e. pregnancy, diabetes mellitus, etc. (see Chapter 3).
2. To note the existence of systemic conditions for which special precautions (e.g. antibiotic prophylaxis) are required to safeguard the patient during periodontal therapy.
3. To note the existence of any transmissible disease which may present a hazard to the clinician, dental surgery staff or other patients.

Examination

A systematic examination should lead to a full diagnosis and reveal the extent and severity of the disease with a view to advising the patient of the treatment options and the likely prognosis.

Gingival inflammation, plaque and calculus

Gingivitis may be recognized by the characteristic appearance of inflammation, such as change of colour from pink to red and enlargement due to oedema or hyperplasia (see Fig. 2.2). Gingival exudate may be evident if the teeth are dried. Bleeding will usually occur when a periodontal probe is run along the soft-tissue wall at the entrance to the gingival pocket. Suppuration, ulceration or swelling may indicate acute inflammation, such as an abscess or ulcerative gingivitis.

A record of plaque and gingivitis should be made at the initial visit and repeated at subsequent appointments to monitor the progress of treatment. Many of the indices which have been devised for this purpose are complex and time-consuming to employ and are, therefore, suitable only for clinical trials. In routine clinical practice, therefore, it is customary merely to record the presence or absence of plaque in contact with the gingivae, and the presence or absence of bleeding from the gingival margin, elicited by a periodontal probe. These assessments are made for each site in the mouth, thereby recording the extent of plaque and gingivitis, but not the quantity of plaque or severity of gingivitis.

An index of gingival health is generally more informative than a plaque index. Some patients may achieve very low plaque indices but may do so only to impress the dentist at the time of appointment. Such patients will not achieve significant improvement of their gingival inflammation index. Nevertheless, gingivitis may sometimes persist, not because of poor home care, but due to the presence of subgingival deposits.

There is great variation between individuals in the tendency for mineralization of plaque. Supragingival calculus is easy to remove, but subgingival calculus is extremely adherent and its presence in large amounts points to a prolonged phase of scaling and root planing.

Finally, one must be wary of forming an impression of attachment levels purely on the amount of plaque and calculus and the severity of gingival inflammation. Severe gingivitis may be present without attachment loss, or attachment loss may be present without gross evidence of gingivitis.

Periodontal probing

The periodontal probe can be used to assess pocket depths and to identify pockets which bleed on probing.

The depth to which the periodontal probe will penetrate beyond the gingival margin depends on:

Factors which influence probing depth
1. The amount of gingival enlargement.
2. The extent of connective tissue attachment loss.
3. The resistance of the tissue to probing, determined by the extent to which gingival collagen has been replaced by inflammatory infiltrate.
4. The size, shape and tip diameter of the probe.
5. Use of the probe – angle of insertion and pressure applied.
6. The presence of obstructions such as subgingival calculus.
7. The patient's reaction to the discomfort of probing.

These factors illustrate why the true depth of the pocket may not be accurately recorded by probing and the expression 'probing depth' is now often used instead of the more traditional 'pocket depth' when referring to the results of an examination with the periodontal probe. Probing depths, nevertheless, may give the best indication of the severity and extent of periodontal disease compared with other clinical or radiographic parameters. Furthermore, the probing depth gives a rough indication of the likely response to treatment because adequate débridement becomes more difficult as probing depths increase. Surgical access is more likely to be required for débridement of deep pockets.

The probing distance from the amelocemental junction to the base of the pocket gives the amount of attachment loss. However, in determining the ultimate prognosis of the tooth, proper consideration must be given to the amount of *residual* supporting tissue, which may be gauged to some extent by mobility tests and by reference to radiographs.

The cardinal sign of a pathological pocket is bleeding on probing, as the instrument breaches the ulcerated and inflamed pocket wall. In patients with untreated periodontal disease, generally, all pockets of around 3 mm and over will bleed on probing. On the other hand, where a long junctional epithelium has formed, consequent upon successful treatment, probing depths of 3–4 mm may be present without eliciting a bleeding response from this healthy but penetrable sulcus. Whereas it is generally accepted that bleeding on probing is the cardinal sign of disease, there is no evidence that the amount of bleeding is related to the rate of attachment loss or to the likelihood of further loss of attachment.

Occlusion, mobility and migration

Various systems exist to classify mobility, based usually on subjective judgements. One system is recommended in Appendix II.

If mobility is present, the occlusion should be checked for premature or interfering contacts and for evidence of food impaction, but a decision on occlusal therapy should, if possible, be delayed until the response to hygiene therapy can be assessed. Mobility in teeth with furcation lesions is usually a late sign and generally indicates a poor prognosis. Such teeth are unlikely to be candidates for root separation techniques, as a further increase in mobility can be anticipated once the 'tripod' or 'bipod' of roots is divided.

Among the many forms of tooth migration, anterior tooth migration is the most unacceptable to the patient. The case history should have established whether parafunctional habits may have been responsible. The occlusion should now be examined for interfering contacts as contributory factors (see Chapter 18). Unfortunately, upper anterior tooth migration is often accompanied by over-eruption of the affected tooth and of its antagonist in the lower arch. Such changes complicate orthodontic treatment.

Mucogingival relationships

The terms 'attached' and 'keratinized' gingiva should be distinguished. Keratinized gingiva is only 'attached' where periosteal or dentogingival attachment exists coronal to the mucogingival line. Thus, marginal bone loss will lead to loss of attached gingiva but not to loss of keratinized gingiva unless there is also recession.

A shallow vestibule or a high fraenal attachment may impair access for adequate plaque control, while a lack of keratinized gingiva may result in mucosal trauma during toothbrushing. Chapter 17 is devoted to the aetiology and management of mucogingival problems.

Furcation lesions

The frequency and extent of furcation lesions are usually underestimated. This may be due to inadequate assessment of root anatomy, reliance on the straight periodontal probe rather than exploration with a curved instrument, and to misinterpretation of radiographs which invariably do not reveal the true extent of involvement. Furcations should be checked carefully so that the feasibility of satisfactory treatment can be assessed. It should be remembered that proximal surface furcation lesions may affect the support of adjacent teeth unless they are separated by a broad interradicular septum.

Generally, the mesial furcation of upper molars is more easily examined from the palatal side, the distal furcation from the buccal. This is because the mesiobuccal root is broader buccopalatally than the distobuccal root and the palatal root is situated distopalatally (see Fig. 13.1).

Radiographs

Radiographs cannot be used to diagnose current periodontal disease since they cannot show whether marginal bone loss is associated with inflamed tissues or with tissues which have been restored to health as a result of successful treatment. Indeed, although a gingival soft-tissue shadow may be visible, radiographs do not reveal pockets.

Radiographs are, however, necessary to assess the proportion of support lost in relation to root length. Periapical radiographs, taken with the 'long cone paralleling' technique, are most useful. Inevitably, however, there are limitations to the use of radiographs in periodontics because of the superimposition of tooth on bone and cortical bone on cancellous bone. Thus, buccal and/or lingual bone margins may be visible interproximally but angular defects and furcation lesions, may be wholly or partially obscured.

The appearance of the crestal bone is a function of X-ray beam angulation and cannot be relied upon as an indicator of disease activity or healing. Indeed, there are no radiographic features which indicate whether disease is progressing or static.

Radiographs will also reveal unerupted teeth, periapical pathology, inadequate endodontic treatment, caries, overhanging margins, etc., which may have a bearing on tooth prognosis or the planning of subsequent restorative treatment.

Study casts

Study casts can be used for assessment of occlusal relationships and treatment options without the patient being present. Proper occlusal analysis is only possible if study casts are accurately mounted on an anatomical articulator, but hand-held casts can provide valuable information and may facilitate the presentation of information to the patient.

Special tests

Pulp vitality tests should be carried out for teeth associated with deep periodontal pockets where pulpitis or pulp necrosis may have resulted from periodontal disease. Vitality tests may also help to distinguish a periapical from a periodontal abscess. In this respect, multirooted teeth require careful interpretation (see Chapter 14).

Haematological investigations such as a full blood count and film are indicated where blood dyscrasias such as neutropenia, leukaemia or thrombocytopenia are suspected.

Diagnosis

Periodontal disease nomenclature is discussed in Chapter 5. For an individual patient, it may be possible to make a diagnosis for the whole dentition which describes the predominant feature. Ideally, however, a tooth-by-tooth diagnosis should be made at the patient's initial examination and again following hygiene therapy.

Patients presenting with significant periodontal disease will require a thorough examination before treatment, and numerous systems exist for recording the results of detailed examination procedures. The chart illustrated in Appendix II has space reserved for recording probing depth measurements for each tooth surface, tooth mobility scores and furcation lesions. The treatment required can be determined for each tooth individually. A detailed assessment of this type is desirable at the patient's first visit and essential after hygiene therapy to determine the need, if any, for more elaborate treatment procedures.

For a simple and rapid method of recording periodontal conditions during a routine dental examination, the reader is referred to Appendix I where the Community Periodontal Index of Treatment Needs (CPITN) is described. Comprehensive examination will, however, be required to select hopeless teeth for extraction, to establish the extent of furcation lesions, to diagnose combined periodontal–endodontic lesions and to evaluate the full extent and significance of mucogingival problems.

Prognosis

Assessment should always be made of prognosis without treatment as well as prognosis for various treatment options. Thus some means are required to determine the likelihood of disease progression.

Much of the periodontal literature in recent years has been concerned with the search for indicators of disease activity as determinants of prognosis and the need for treatment. Attention has focused on microbiological, immunological and biochemical characteristics of periodontal diseases, but there is still little prospect of a test with the necessary criteria of sensitivity, specificity and cost effectiveness.

It would appear that bleeding on probing combined with a history of attachment loss is currently the best predictor of future attachment loss, but when or how quickly this will occur is impossible to determine. The absence of bleeding on probing or the absence of attachment loss suggests a *low* probability of periodontal breakdown in the near future.

For ongoing disease, it will be apparent that prognosis is dependent on the adequacy of diagnosis and the quality of treatment, including home care and recall maintenance.

Rationale of treatment

The main purpose of this chapter is to seek answers to the following questions:

- What happens if periodontal disease is left untreated?
- How successful is treatment?
- How much time and effort are involved?
- Who should receive treatment?
- What are the objectives?
- What is the nature of the healing process?
- What form does treatment take?

Consequences of periodontal disease

Gingivitis and periodontitis, as described in Chapter 5, are very common, both conditions affecting most individuals by adulthood. Periodontitis tends to be progressive and ultimately gives rise to 20–30% of all extractions in countries which offer good access to dental care.

While tooth loss may be the ultimate consequence of untreated periodontal disease, it is not the only one: distress caused by swollen, bleeding gums, bad taste, bad breath and occlusal instability can occur long before patients are faced with the prospect of extractions.

Effectiveness of periodontal treatment

Numerous clinical trials and retrospective studies have documented the effectiveness of various forms of treatment in controlling periodontal disease, while also revealing that, among patients with severe periodontitis – those most susceptible to dental plaque infection – 25% of treated sites, on average, continue to bleed on probing. Continuing or recurrent disease is usually attributable to incomplete root débridement or failure of daily plaque control.

Time required for treatment

Clearly, the time spent in treatment will depend on the extent and severity of the disease. The proper management of *severe* periodontitis is certainly labour intensive, and the data below, which are drawn from the literature, reflect the time required for a typical course of treatment.

Time to treat severe periodontitis
- Education and instruction   60–90 minutes per patient
- Scaling and root planing   5–10 minutes per tooth
- Surgery   10–12 minutes per tooth
- Maintenance care   120–240 minutes per year

Case selection

Patients' treatment needs must be assessed within a context of available resources. This applies whether treatment is hospital-based or focused in general or specialist practice, and whether it is publicly or privately funded. It is unrealistic, therefore, to seek to eradicate all signs of disease in all patients.

At one extreme, attachment loss and bleeding on probing in an adolescent or young adult, with relatively good plaque control, are a sign of poor prognosis, and treatment should be instituted without delay. Many patients, however, will have minor amounts of plaque and gingivitis throughout their lives and little evidence of destructive changes. For them, the requirement for periodontal treatment recedes as they become older, untroubled by symptoms and without significant attachment loss. Low-risk patients in younger age groups, however, can only be recognized as such when they attend for periodic review, and only if a record of periodontal conditions is kept. The onset of symptoms, or an increase in bleeding on probing, probing depth, recession or tooth mobility should signal the need for more concerted treatment. In theory, attachment levels can also be monitored, but this would be extremely time-consuming and would in any case be subject to considerable measurement error.

Objectives of treatment
Relief of symptoms

Relief from symptoms contributes to the patient's sense of personal well-being, and is, therefore, an important objective always worth pursuing even in those cases where complete restoration of periodontal health is unattainable. 'Success' in periodontal therapy should not be measured only by the yardstick of restored periodontal health.

Restoration of periodontal health

Periodontal health can be defined as absence of gingival inflammation and progressive breakdown of the supporting tissues of the tooth. At the dentogingival junction, there will be a *physiological gingival sulcus*, recognizable clinically by the absence of bleeding on probing, and this, where possible, should be the treatment goal. However, acceptance of a lesser standard of improved periodontal health – an overall reduction in the frequency and depth of bleeding pockets – is, in many cases, necessary.

If elaborate treatment procedures are required which are dependent on good oral hygiene, these are deferred until initial progress has been assessed; patients who maintain a positive attitude will, thereby, achieve the highest standards of periodontal health.

Restoration and maintenance of function and aesthetics

Diminished chewing function may result, not only from tooth loss, but also from excessive tooth mobility or tooth migration. A migrated anterior tooth may also be unaesthetic. Treatment cannot be considered complete until such teeth are restored to function and stabilized within the arch. Occasionally, gross gingival overgrowth may be present and, as well as being unaesthetic, the gingival surface may be traumatized by opposing teeth. In such cases, periodontal treatment should include measures to restore function and aesthetics.

Structural changes after treatment

The formation of a physiological sulcus is a feature common to the healing of all inflammatory periodontal lesions, but the structural reorganization of the underlying connective tissues will depend on the damage previously inflicted.

Treatment of gingivitis

Figure 7.1 illustrates a limited gingivitis (Fig. 7.1(a)) and the structure of the gingiva (Fig. 7.1(b)) once healing has taken place

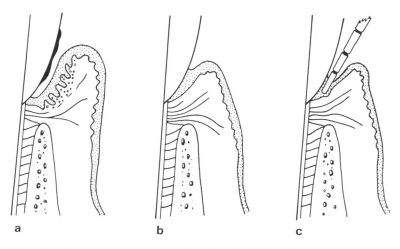

a   b   c

Fig. 7.1 Treatment of gingivitis. (a) Gingivitis. (b) Normal healthy periodontium after treatment. (c) 'Normal' probing depth after treatment.

following removal of plaque and calculus. The pocket epithelium undergoes transition to junctional epithelium which forms an attachment to the adjacent tooth surface. The inflammatory infiltrate is gradually replaced by maturing collagen fibres which eventually become organized into functionally orientated bundles. Clinically these healing events are manifested as a change to a uniform pink colour, a reduction in gingival bulk and the formation of a physiological gingival sulcus with a 'normal' probing depth of 0.5–2.5 mm (Fig. 7.1(c)). Gingivitis then, from both a clinical and histological viewpoint, is reversible. Tissues are restored not just to health but also to normality. This may necessitate surgical excision if gross fibrous enlargement has occurred.

Treatment of periodontitis

Periodontitis is characterized by loss of connective tissue attachment (Figs 7.2(a) and 7.3(a)). Successful treatment depends on the removal of plaque, calculus and contaminated cementum accompanied by very good plaque control. This leads to elimination of inflammation with *repair* but not *regeneration* of the supporting tissues. Similar results may be achieved with or without surgical access in suitably selected cases. Following subgingival scaling and root planing, remnants of pocket epithelium will be trans-

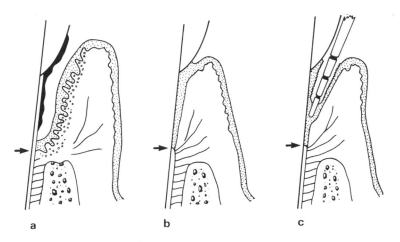

a   b   c

Fig. 7.2 Treatment of periodontitis (suprabony pocket): arrows indicate connective tissue attachment levels. (a) Periodontitis with suprabony pocket. (b) Reduced healthy periodontium after treatment. (c) Gain in clinical attachment after treatment.

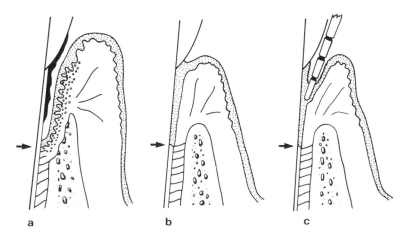

a   b   c

Fig. 7.3 Treatment of periodontitis (infrabony pocket): arrows represent connective tissue attachment levels. (a) Periodontitis with infrabony pocket. (b) Reduced healthy periodontium with bone-fill after treatment. (c) Gain in clinical attachment after treatment.

formed into junctional epithelium which will cover the tooth surface down to the base of the original pocket (Figs 7.2(b) and 7.3(b)). Even if the pocket lining is surgically excised, such is the rapidity of epithelial cell migration that the entire area of denuded root becomes covered with junctional epithelium before other tissue cells in the vicinity have colonized any part of the exposed root. The junctional epithelium forms a long epithelial attachment. In the underlying connective tissues, the inflammatory infiltrate will be replaced by collagen but the junctional epithelium will, of course, form a barrier to new fibre attachment.

There will be no increase in crestal bone height. Indeed a slight loss may occur, especially if surgery is performed.

Some angular bone defects, particularly those with three bone walls, may exhibit bone-fill within the boundaries of the defect (Fig. 7.3(b)). It should be noted that bone-fill of angular defects is not accompanied by new connective tissue attachment. Instead, the underlying root surface will be lined with junctional epithelium (Fig. 7.3(b)).

The structural changes described above involve healing with a long junctional epithelium. An alternative approach to the treatment of periodontitis uses surgery, not just to gain access to root surface deposits, but also to 'eliminate' the soft-tissue and hard-tissue pocket walls to produce a dentogingival attachment of normal dimensions and with a limited epithelial component. This approach is based on the belief that, should treatment fail following a period of unsatisfactory plaque control, the pathological pockets which form will be relatively shallow and, therefore, comparatively easy to re-instrument.

Clinically, following successful treatment of periodontitis, the gingiva should appear uniformly pink and firm, and some gingival recession will inevitably have occurred, more so after surgery. Tooth mobility may have decreased. Most significantly, with the formation of a physiological gingival sulcus, there should be no bleeding on probing. There will be a reduction in probing depth, although, if a long junctional epithelium has formed, it may be possible, with a probe inserted into the sulcus, to displace the gingival tissue relatively easily and record probing depths which are greater than 'normal'. The magnitude of the reduction in clinical pocket depth depends on the extent of gingival recession and the gain in clinical attachment, if any.

Attachment gain

Figures 7.2 and 7.3 show that treatment of periodontitis does not result in an improvement in connective tissue attachment level

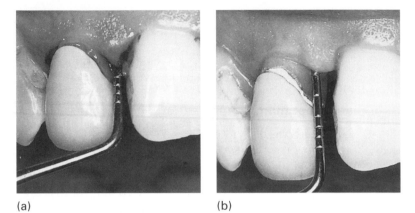

(a)   (b)

Fig. 7.4 Treatment of periodontitis: (a) before; and (b) after treatment. Clinical pocket depth has been reduced from 6 mm to 3 mm. There has been 1-mm recession and a 2-mm gain in clinical attachment (using the lateral incisor crown margin as a fixed reference point against which attachment change may be measured).

(arrowed). The connective tissue attachment level – the level on the root at which the most coronal fibres are attached – can be precisely identified only by histology. However, in the presence of periodontitis, it corresponds roughly to the base of the pocket and so can be identified by probing. After healing, however, because of the improved gingival tone and bone-fill, if any, penetration of the probe will be reduced, giving an apparent gain in attachment. The magnitude of this clinical attachment gain in Figures 7.2(c) and 7.3(c) corresponds to the distance between the arrow (formerly the base of the pocket) and the probe tip. As a general rule, the deeper the pocket, the greater the gain in clinical attachment (Fig. 7.4). It should also be noted that gain in *clinical attachment* is possible even when treatment has induced some loss of *connective tissue attachment*; the resistance to probing after treatment in these cases may mask an underlying true loss of attachment due to instrumentation trauma.

Treatment modalities

Dental health education and instruction

Plaque forms continuously and the object of oral hygiene instruction is to advise the patient how plaque may be successfully removed with a frequency sufficient to prevent pathological effects arising from recurrent plaque accumulation. Motivation is an essential factor in establishing a pattern of behaviour which will make the patient independent of professional support.

Provision of optimum conditions for plaque control

Dental health education and oral hygiene instruction are essential components of periodontal treatment, but so too is the elimination of factors whose presence inhibits adequate self-performed plaque control. These factors include supragingival calculus, malpositioned or badly restored teeth and unfavourable gingival contours or mucogingival relationships.

Subgingival scaling and root planing

Subgingival débridement is required once pathological pockets have formed and their bacterial contents are either calcified or beyond the reach of personal hygiene measures. The deeper the pocket, however, the less effective will this treatment be and the greater the need for surgical intervention.

Accordingly, the approach to pocket therapy, recommended in this text and discussed in more detail in Chapters 9, 10 and 11, is as follows: treatment should commence with a phase of hygiene therapy (dental health education, oral hygiene instruction, scaling and root planing) which should proceed until the patient reaches his peak level of plaque control and all accessible subgingival deposits have been removed; after a healing interval of 4–6 weeks, the patient is re-examined and, if pathological pockets, i.e. pockets which bleed or exude pus on probing, persist at sites of perfect plaque control, surgical intervention should be considered. The success with which root surface irritants can be completely removed from within deep pockets will largely be determined by the clinician's skill and experience, but as a very rough guide, the following outcomes can usually be expected:

- Pockets no more than 3 mm deep should always be amenable to treatment by non-surgical débridement.
- At pocket depths of about 4–5 mm, complete non-surgical débridement should always be attempted. Success will depend to some extent on the skill of the clinician. Dental hygienists and periodontists, for example, should anticipate a successful outcome in the great majority of cases.

- Pockets deeper than 5 mm are often unresponsive to non-surgical débridement. In favourable circumstances, however, where the operator is adequately skilled and access is good, complete healing of deep pockets frequently occurs. Persistent pockets require surgical intervention, subject to the establishment of good oral hygiene.

Experienced clinicians may be able to predict at the patient's initial visit which jaw segments can be treated adequately by a non-surgical approach and which segments are likely to require surgical intervention. In the latter case, subgingival instrumentation may be curtailed once the gross subgingival deposits have been removed. Subject to the establishment of good plaque control, treatment may then be completed surgically without delay, sparing the patient a protracted phase of non-surgical root instrumentation with little expectation of success. Of course, even when surgical intervention appears unavoidable, gross subgingival deposits must first be removed. This will reduce the level of inflammation and improve tissue consistency, thereby permitting improved visibility and better tissue handling during surgery.

Surgical treatment

Severe gingival overgrowth or unsatisfactory mucogingival relationships may require surgical intervention, either to facilitate self-performed plaque control or for cosmetic reasons. The principal use of surgery, however, is in the treatment of advanced periodontitis where the foremost objective is the provision of access for more effective root instrumentation. Whatever technique of surgery is chosen, it is essential that satisfactory gingival contours are produced and it may, therefore, be necessary to remove bone and excise or reposition apically the soft tissue. Wherever possible, the full potential for repair should be exploited by preserving bone and replacing soft tissue to give the results depicted in Figures 7.2(b) and 7.3(b).

It is apparent that surgical treatment of periodontitis is reserved for patients with comparatively advanced disease, i.e. for patients who have shown the greatest susceptibility to plaque infection. It is, therefore, not surprising that a large number of carefully controlled clinical studies have demonstrated a high rate of recurrence where surgery was not supported by a long-term programme of effective home care.

Antimicrobial chemotherapy

Antiplaque mouthwashes may help to inhibit supragingival plaque formation, but none are without side-effects. Chlorhexidine, for example, stains teeth and fillings and causes disturbances of taste. In recent years new treatment strategies involving topical and systemic chemotherapy have been suggested, as adjuncts to scaling and root planing, for the management of chronic periodontitis. These are discussed in Chapter 16.

Maintenance care

A phase of maintenance care should follow the conclusion of active treatment regardless of whether surgery has been carried out. Good oral hygiene is just as important for the continuing success of non-surgical treatment as it is for surgical therapy.

At the completion of therapy it should be possible for the patient to have access to all sites at which plaque will form. Nevertheless, reinforcement of oral hygiene instruction at frequent intervals is essential. Furthermore, supragingival calculus deposits may continue to form and must be removed. The subject of recall maintenance is discussed in greater detail in Chapter 19.

8

Treatment planning

The *general aim* of treatment should be to satisfy the patient's functional and aesthetic requirements within the limits of available resources with a significantly improved prognosis. This will often entail a degree of compromise.

Patients differ in motivation, manual dexterity and availability for treatment. These factors must be taken into account, albeit somewhat subjectively, so that the aims of the operator and expectations of the patient are correlated as closely as possible before treatment begins.

Periodontal treatment cannot be divorced from other dental procedures, and so an overall treatment for the patient must be planned. Study casts and radiographs are invaluable to supplement clinical examination, to facilitate discussion with the patient and as pretreatment records.

Phases of treatment

It is usually convenient to divide the treatment plan into a series of phases. This has the advantage of setting a number of goals and of imparting a sense of achievement for both clinician and patient as each goal is accomplished. The following programme should be seen as a framework within which the precise sequence may be altered or certain elements run concurrently.

1. Relief of acute symptoms.
2. Infection control
   a) Hygiene therapy
   b) Treatment of gross caries and pulp symptoms
   c) Extraction of hopeless posterior teeth.
3. Reassessment and definitive planning.
4. Corrective treatment
   a) Root canal therapy
   b) Orthodontic therapy
   c) Occlusal therapy

    d) Temporization
    e) Periodontal surgery
    f) Fixed and removable prosthodontics.
  5. Recall maintenance.

(1) Relief of acute symptoms

This may be a most rewarding way of gaining a patient's confidence and is usually essential before he can be expected to absorb further information or make decisions about less pressing matters (see Chapter 20).

(2) Infection control

(a) **Hygiene therapy**. This will include dental health education and oral hygiene instruction, correction of local predisposing factors, scaling, root planing and polishing (see Chapters 9 and 10).

Patients should be encouraged to appreciate that improvement in symptoms owes much to their self-performed oral hygiene measures. Nevertheless, to achieve good plaque control, plaque retention factors, such as calculus and restoration overhangs must first be removed. It may also be possible to modify the design of partial dentures by trimming the denture base away from gingival margins. Patients should have detailed denture hygiene instructions and should normally be advised to leave dentures out overnight.

Once supragingival plaque is under control, subgingival scaling and root planing should proceed, and be continued until all accessible deposits have been removed.

The number of visits for hygiene therapy will clearly depend on the extent and severity of periodontal disease. When several visits are necessary, the interval between appointments should be as short as possible consistent with the rate of acquisition of plaque control skills, so that a good healing momentum can be established and maintained. This is the most efficient way to reduce the pool of pathogenic organisms and there is some evidence that re-infection of treated areas may be less likely to occur if treatment proceeds rapidly.

(b) **Treatment of gross caries and pulp symptoms**. This should be carried out to assess the feasibility of retaining and restoring such teeth and to avoid complications at a later stage.

(c) **Extraction of hopeless posterior teeth**. Teeth which exhibit very advanced periodontal breakdown should be extracted. As a general rule, extractions, once decided upon, should be carried out early in treatment to facilitate healing of the periodontal tissues of adjacent teeth. This recommendation applies particularly to posterior teeth which rarely require immediate replacement with a denture.

(3) Reassessment and definitive planning

Timing of reassessment. Following hygiene therapy, a time lapse of a few months is theoretically desirable before reassessment, to give some indication of the likelihood of long-term maintenance of oral hygiene by the patient. However, for practical purposes it is desirable to proceed with treatment planning as soon as maximal resolution of inflammation has taken place, about 4–6 weeks after the completion of hygiene therapy.

Success of hygiene therapy. Patients who require no further treatment should be enrolled on a programme of recall maintenance. Where 'corrective treatment' is required, the definitive treatment plan will be influenced by the response to hygiene therapy, this being an important prognostic indicator.

Assessment of plaque control. Planning is usually easier when motivation and cooperation are not in doubt. However, in practice, many patients, through lack of motivation or manual dexterity, fail to achieve satisfactory levels of plaque control, and it is consequently more difficult to arrive at a satisfactory treatment plan. The patient's aesthetic and functional expectations may need to be reduced and fulfilled by simpler forms of treatment. It may also be necessary to acknowledge that deterioration is likely and advise the patient accordingly.

Case assessment and presentation. The periodontal charting (Appendix II) should be completed with details of probing depths, mobility and furcation lesions, and comparison with earlier charting will give some indication of progress. Scrutiny of the chart, study casts and radiographs will allow decisions to be made about the wisdom of retaining teeth affected by advanced lesions, the need for surgery and the design of partial prostheses. Frequently, a number of options will be available and these must be discussed with the patient so that a step-by-step, detailed treatment plan may be formulated.

Surgical intervention. Surgery is justified only for patients with good plaque control and any temptation to 'improve' a periodontium surgically and work on plaque control later must be resisted, particularly as research has shown that rapid loss of attachment can be expected if plaque accumulation occurs after surgery.

Occlusal function. At this stage it must be decided which teeth are to be retained and an attempt should be made to maintain opposing teeth in occlusal function. A complete lower denture opposed by natural upper teeth is rarely acceptable and considerable effort should be made to avoid this: the relatively poor support and retention of a complete lower denture, opposed by natural upper teeth, may result in mucosal trauma and accelerated resorption of the lower residual alveolar ridge.

Tooth replacement. It must also be decided whether it is necessary (or desirable) to replace missing teeth, and the possible designs of bridgework or partial denture should be considered at this stage.

Planning for edentulousness. Many patients will require some planning for edentulousness. Thus, it may be necessary to offset the deterioration which will result from wearing a transitional partial denture when oral hygiene is poor, against the advantages of a period of adaptation before a complete denture becomes inevitable.

(4) Corrective treatment

(a) Root canal therapy. Where an infected pulp communicates with a marginal periodontal lesion, endodontic treatment should be undertaken in the first instance. Attempts at periodontal treatment will otherwise be frustrated because of leakage from the infected pulp space. Moreover, where the periodontal 'pocket' is no more than a sinus tract, arising from the apex or from an accessory or lateral root canal, complete resolution of the periodontal lesion may be achieved by root canal therapy alone (see Chapter 14).

Root canal therapy will be required for teeth with furcation lesions prior to root separation. This subject is considered in greater detail in Chapter 13.

(b) Orthodontic therapy. In the adult dentition affected by periodontitis, tooth migration is a common occurrence which is rarely limited to the movement of a single tooth in one direction. Instead, there may be a complex mixture of bodily movement, tipping and rotation with secondary movement of adjacent and opposing teeth. Realignment, therefore, frequently requires elaborate orthodontic treatment. On the other hand, it can often be accomplished in a relatively short time because of the reduction in supporting tissues which has taken place.

Orthodontic therapy for the periodontal patient may also be indicated: to allow the achievement of a normal lip seal where protruding upper incisors are affected by 'mouthbreathing gingivitis'; to relieve deep traumatic overbite; to realign teeth partially excluded from the arch and suffering gingival recession as a result of this; to correct tooth malalignment caused by severe fibrous gingival overgrowth; and to 'upright' tilted molars.

Orthodontic treatment for teeth affected by periodontitis should be carried out only after thorough subgingival débridement to avoid the risk of an acute periodontal abscess when the pocket wall is compressed by the plaque-infected root surface.

A very important consideration, prior to any orthodontic treatment, and particularly for teeth with reduced periodontal support, is the means by which these teeth may be permanently retained in their new position. Permanent retention may be more difficult to provide than the orthodontic treatment itself.

Anterior tooth migration, deep traumatic overbite and splinting after tooth movement are discussed in greater detail in Chapter 18.

(c) Occlusal therapy. Tooth mobility is often less apparent following the completion of hygiene therapy, but occlusal therapy may still be required to improve tooth stability and involves occlusal adjustment or splinting (see Chapter 18). Teeth which have been subjected to orthodontic movement will usually require splinting. Likewise, it is occasionally necessary to splint teeth which are exceptionally mobile to avoid the risk of accidental avulsion during or immediately after surgery. Splinting may also be advisable where very mobile teeth cause discomfort.

(d) Temporization. Where it is anticipated that bridgework will ultimately replace a removable partial denture, it is often helpful to carry out tooth preparation as far as possible and fit a temporary bridge prior to surgical intervention. By eliminating the partial denture, postoperative healing will be improved. It will frequently be necessary, however, to adjust the cervical margins and take the final impression of the crown preparations after surgery to take account of the surgically-induced recession. Where a fixed bridge is intended principally to stabilize mobile teeth, presurgical temporization will have the added advantage of facilitating the surgical procedure.

(e) Periodontal surgery. If pathological pockets persist after thorough tooth instrumentation at sites of good plaque control, surgical intervention should be considered to complete the process of root débridement. Furthermore, surgery may occasionally be required to reduce gingival bulk or improve gingival contour, to create new attached gingiva where mucogingival problems exist and to increase clinical crown length in order to facilitate restorative procedures or improve artificial crown retention.

(f) Fixed and removable prosthodontics. The highest quality operative dentistry can be carried out only on teeth with good gingival conditions where gingival fluid flow and bleeding in response to minor trauma will be minimal. Gingival retraction, where necessary, can be carried out easily and this will result in better impressions, better-fitting crowns and less risk of subsequent gingival irritation or recession. Plastic restorations may be placed dry. The increase in crown length which results from reduction of marginal oedema and surgery may make available additional undercut areas for partial denture retention.

Replacement of missing teeth is not invariably necessary but may be required for aesthetic or functional reasons or as part of a transition to complete dentures. It may be desirable, also, to prevent further tipping, drifting or over-eruption, or to redistribute masticatory forces and achieve stabilization of hypermobile teeth.

Where appropriate, a well-designed bridge is almost invariably preferable to a well-designed partial denture. Indeed, the latter may have an adverse effect on prognosis by enhancing plaque accumulation.

A partial denture can only be expected to improve the prognosis for remaining teeth if oral and denture hygiene are excellent, and if the denture makes a positive contribution towards more even distribution of occlusal forces, so limiting mobility or tendency to migrate. On the other hand, it may be advisable to provide partial dentures when further deterioration and tooth loss appear inevitable, in order that the patient may have some denture experience before provision of complete dentures. If possible, allowance should be made in the denture design for further tooth loss.

There are many patients in whom a premolar-to-premolar occlusion (shortened dental arch) is acceptable both functionally and cosmetically. In considering whether a shortened dental arch should be extended by a prosthesis, one should weigh the risks of reduced molar support (increasing mobility, migration or attrition of anterior teeth) against the potentially harmful effects of a partial denture on the remaining dentition.

Definitive restorative treatment should not be undertaken until optimum periodontal conditions are achieved and maintained.

(5) Recall maintenance

This is essential for a good prognosis and must be seen as a long-term requirement. Recall maintenance is discussed in detail in Chapter 19.

9

The control of dental plaque

In the periodontal context, the purpose of dental health education is to establish behaviour which will prevent significant pathological effects of recurrent plaque accumulation and make the patient as independent as possible of professional support. This involves a number of related processes including the setting of objectives for dental health and treatment, informal and formal health education, and instruction in plaque control.

Dental health education

A discussion of health education theory is beyond the scope of this text. Nevertheless, the provision of effective dental health education is no less important than the clinical skills required to treat periodontal disease, and some practical guidelines are listed below:

1. Use terminology and language appropriate to the patient's education and background.
2. Avoid giving offence, when commenting on poor oral hygiene habits.
3. Explanatory leaflets may be useful but should be supported by a personalized account of periodontal disease, the nature of treatment and prognosis.
4. Plaque, gingivitis, bleeding and pockets can easily be demonstrated in the patient's mouth. This will encourage self-assessment which is especially valuable when the maintenance phase is reached and visits to the dentist become less frequent.
5. Disclosing agents may be useful initially, but should not be relied upon for long-term maintenance of oral hygiene.
6. Help the patient to recognize the benefits of prevention. The avoidance of tooth loss and financial expense, and the preservation of appearance are obvious goals. However, in some cases, an appeal to the patient's social awareness, for

example the desire to have fresh breath, may prove more successful.

7. Do not build up false hopes which cannot be fulfilled, or create unfounded fears which may arouse feelings of resentment. Learning is more satisfactory in an atmosphere of trust and security.
8. Periodontal treatment is frequently protracted and patients need constant encouragement to maintain their motivational drive. This encouragement can only be given by setting short-term goals, such as a reduction in plaque score or bleeding points.
9. Stress every positive result at follow-up appointments and watch out for signs of discouragement.

Oral hygiene instruction

Frequency of tooth cleaning

The prevention and treatment of chronic periodontal disease involves the thorough removal of plaque, sufficiently frequently to prevent pathological effects arising from recurrent plaque formation. Patients should, therefore, carry out thorough plaque removal once or twice daily according to their professionally assessed individual needs.

The thoroughness of plaque removal is important, since careless tooth cleaning will result in certain tooth surfaces consistently being missed, and patients should be discouraged from cleaning more frequently/less thoroughly.

Toothbrushing

The brush. Most adults should use a brush head approximately one inch long; a smaller head is appropriate for children. Multitufted, soft-filament nylon brushes are most widely accepted at the present time.

Toothpaste. The abrasive property of toothpaste contributes to the removal of plaque by brushes and other aids, keeps the pellicle layer thin and prevents the accumulation of surface stains. Most toothpastes also contain fluoride, antimicrobials or anticalculus agents which may have plaque- or calculus-inhibitory effects. Among the newer formulations, toothpastes containing triclosan, with a copolymer or with zinc citrate, show promise as antiplaque agents.

Technique. The Bass technique, or some modification of it, is regarded as the most efficient (Fig. 9.1). However, there is no

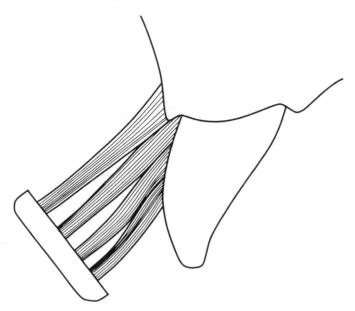

Fig. 9.1 The Bass method of toothbrushing. The bristles are directed into the gingival sulcus at 45° angle to the long axis of the teeth and the brush is activated with a short back-and-forth vibrating motion.

point in insisting that patients conform to a particular technique if brushing is already effective, unless there is evidence of toothbrush trauma. Furthermore, advice to brush for a longer period might be more beneficial to many patients than dwelling unduly on a particular technique.

Vigorous brushing may cause gingival abrasion, gingival recession and tooth abrasion, usually most pronounced in the canine and premolar regions. Toothbrush trauma may be minimized by: using a *medium-soft* filament brush; minimal use of toothpaste; avoiding a forceful scrubbing action; and shifting the brushing emphasis to the lingual surfaces, which are often comparatively neglected.

Special brushes. In certain cases, where patient motivation seems adequate, the use of special brushes such as the single-tufted brush ('interspace brush') may be recommended: to clean malaligned teeth and teeth affected by localized gingival recession; to clean the proximal surfaces of teeth adjacent to a saddle area; to clean the distal surface of the last molar tooth; and, as an adjunct to interdental woodsticks, to compensate for the failure of the latter to remove plaque from lingual embrasures.

Electric toothbrushes may be helpful to physically or mentally handicapped patients, or to those responsible for assisting others with toothcleaning. The new generation of electric toothbrushes with rotating tufts would appear to be more effective, particularly at cleaning interdental embrasures, than traditional electric brushes.

Neither manual nor electric toothbrushes will remove plaque from proximal surface contact areas. The use of manual or, indeed, electric interdental cleaning devices is, therefore, essential.

Interdental cleaning

Periodontal health is seldom achieved without the use of interdental cleaning aids such as dental floss, interdental brushes or woodsticks. Efficiently used, floss is more effective than woodsticks at removing plaque from proximal surfaces, subgingival surfaces and from lingual embrasures. The use of floss, however, is time-consuming and calls for a degree of motivation and dexterity not found in all individuals. In general, the use of woodsticks takes less time than floss, calls for less manual dexterity and, consequently, may require slightly less motivation. It may, in some cases, be preferable to accept regular use of woodsticks than infrequent use of floss. On the other hand, the woodstick is effective only where sufficient interdental space is available to accommodate it.

If any proximal attachment loss has occurred, the gingival recession, which will inevitably occur with treatment, should allow interdental brushes ('bottle brushes') to be used in preference to floss or woodsticks. In these cases, although the embrasure spaces may be filled by the papilla prior to treatment, an interdental space should appear and gradually enlarge as plaque removal by scaling and flossing gives rise to tissue shrinkage. This will allow the floss to be replaced by an interdental brush. Interdental brushes, furthermore, are *essential* where interdental recession has progressed to expose proximal root furrows, which cannot be adequately cleaned by floss or sticks (Fig. 9.2).

Interdental brushes are available in a range of different sizes, and some patients may require two or three different sizes of brush to suit variations in the size of their interdental spaces. For each space, the largest brush to fit comfortably should be chosen.

Young children are unlikely to possess either the manual dexterity or the motivation to practise interdental cleaning. However, interdental cleaning should certainly be recommended once most of the permanent dentition is established in

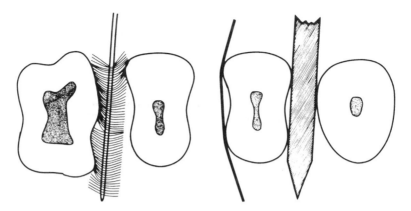

Fig. 9.2 Interdental aids: failure of woodpoints and dental floss to clean proximal root furrows, compared with the interdental brush, which enters these root surface concavities when correctly angulated.

the early teenage years. At this age, interdental gingival recession is unlikely to have occurred and dental floss will be the only suitable aid.

While toothbrushing is invigorating and, therefore, well accepted, most patients find little incentive for interdental cleaning, which is comparatively difficult and time-consuming, whatever means are employed. Nonetheless, thorough *daily* interdental cleaning is essential for periodontal patients and also advisable as a preventive measure for individuals with no history of periodontal problems. The establishment and maintenance of a good interdental cleaning habit is the principal goal of dental health education and instruction for periodontal patients.

Mouthwashes

Antimicrobial mouthwashes which have been tested *in vivo* and/or *in vitro* include bisbiguanide antiseptics, quaternary ammonium compounds, phenolic compounds, amino alcohols, enzymes aimed at disruption of plaque or potentiation of salivary antibacterial activity, fluoride or metallic ions, such as zinc and tin, natural antiseptics, such as sanguinarine, and surface active agents present in pre-brushing rinses. However, although plaque- and gingivitis-inhibitory effects have been demonstrated for some agents, these are, in most cases, of insufficient magnitude to justify their widespread adoption.

The most effective chemical antimicrobial agent available at the present time is chlorhexidine gluconate. Chlorhexidine is a cationic bisbiguanide antiseptic which possesses the property of adsorption to oral surfaces, notably enamel, where it exerts a prolonged antimicrobial action. It has a fairly broad antimicrobial spectrum.

Used twice daily (either 10 ml of a 0.2% solution or 15 ml of a 0.12% solution), it will effectively prevent plaque accumulation and gingivitis. However, when used as a mouthwash, it will not penetrate subgingivally and is unlikely to have any worthwhile effect where gingival or periodontal pockets are present. Furthermore, it has an unpleasant taste, interferes with taste appreciation, and discolours teeth and restorations. Less common side-effects, usually after longer use, are mucosal erosion, which is concentration dependent and, very rarely, parotid enlargement. These factors limit the periodontal use of chlorhexidine mouthwash to situations where mechanical plaque control is difficult or impossible.

Periodontal uses of chlorhexidine
1. Postoperative management of periodontal wounds.
2. Patients with painful gingival lesions.
3. Patients with intermaxillary fixation.
4. After acute necrotizing ulcerative gingivitis, when sensitivity and poor gingival contours inhibit mechanical tooth cleaning.
5. Long-term management of periodontal health in handicapped individuals or medically compromised patients.

Chlorhexidine mouthwash used during the initial phase of hygiene therapy will mask the effects of personal mechanical plaque control, and will make proper evaluation of the patient's efforts impossible. Use of chlorhexidine during hygiene therapy is, therefore, advised only on the rare occasion when gingivitis is so severe that effective mechanical oral hygiene is impossible, and then the drug should be withdrawn at the earliest opportunity.

Concluding remarks

Oral hygiene instruction will rarely produce the desired result after only one session, and many visits may be necessary, during which patients should demonstrate their toothcleaning skills, while the clinician observes and offers help where necessary.

Visits for oral hygiene instruction should continue until the peak level of performance has been reached.

Personal mechanical plaque control, and indeed chemical antiplaque agents, can prevent gingivitis and may resolve inflammation in its early stages. Their effectiveness in preventing the extension of established periodontitis is, however, very limited. Professional subgingival cleaning is, therefore, an essential part of treatment where pockets are present.

Scaling and root planing

Effective scaling and root planing are fundamental to the success of all aspects of periodontal treatment. Expertise in this field is essential for all those involved in the management of periodontal disease. Much of this chapter applies equally to the scaling and root planing procedures which accompany most forms of surgical therapy, although the comments which follow are primarily about non-surgical débridement.

Aims and objectives

The aims and objectives of tooth surface instrumentation are:

Aims and objectives
1. To remove supragingival accretions leaving a smooth and polished surface which will facilitate rapid and simple day-to-day plaque control by the patient.
2. To remove subgingival root surface irritants, i.e. plaque, calculus and pathologically altered cementum.
3. To obtain healing of the adjacent soft tissues with formation of new epithelial attachment and a physiological gingival sulcus.

Scaling and root planing are fully effective only at surfaces which are readily accessible to instrumentation, and at these sites there is no certain magnitude of initial probing depth beyond which non-surgical instrumentation is ineffective, provided sufficient skill is exercised. Even when subgingival instrumentation is incomplete, and when healing of the pocket wall is not achieved, the progress of periodontal disease may still be retarded by the effects of débridement until a periodontopathic flora becomes re-established.

Terminology

Scaling. The term 'scaling' refers to the physical removal of tooth surface accretions, notably plaque, calculus and stained pellicle.

Root planing involves the removal of pathologically altered cementum and smoothing of the root surface. This process should also remove plaque and calculus which have become embedded in surface irregularities. The degree of root smoothness which is achieved may not be of biological importance but it gives the best clinical indication that calculus and altered cementum have been removed. The exposure of root dentine, although not intended, may be unavoidable.

Scaling and root planing are best considered as a single treatment procedure since scaling inevitably removes some cementum, and root planing will remove embedded plaque and calculus deposits.

Curettage. Subgingival scaling and root planing are sometimes referred to as 'root curettage'. The term 'subgingival curettage' is reserved for scraping and removal of soft tissue from within the pocket. A certain amount of subgingival curettage is unavoidable during scaling and root planing, particularly when curettes are used. Nevertheless, it has been shown that deliberate subgingival curettage is not a worthwhile procedure, since the results achieved by scaling and root planing with subgingival curettage are no better than those obtained by scaling and root planing alone.

Detection of calculus

Supragingival calculus is easily identified when present in large deposits, and trace amounts can be readily visualized by drying the teeth with an air syringe.

Superficial deposits of subgingival calculus may be identified to some extent by distending the pocket orifice with a flat plastic instrument, or by gently blowing air into the pocket. More deeply located deposits can be detected only by probing, using a fine pointed probe or a fine ball-ended probe (CPITN probe).

Radiographs are unreliable for calculus detection since only large radio-opaque deposits will be visible, and then only on proximal surfaces.

Treatment procedures

Supragingival instrumentation

Generally, it is advisable to complete the supragingival scaling in the first appointment to facilitate the patient's personal plaque control. All accessible surfaces should then be polished with a fine abrasive polishing paste to reduce surface roughness as far as possible, so minimizing subsequent plaque accumulation. Polishing pastes which are sufficiently abrasive to remove stains will also remove tooth substance and leave a rough surface. Coarse pastes should, therefore, be used only on surfaces where stain removal is necessary, and this should be followed by a polish with a fine-particle paste. At the following visit, 1–2 weeks later, substantial resolution of superficial inflammation should be apparent.

Subgingival instrumentation

The approach to subgingival débridement will largely depend on the distribution and depth of pockets. Subgingival instrumentation, ideally, should not be initiated until the patient is capable of performing adequate plaque control. It is likely to be much more time-consuming than supragingival scaling, in view of the greater hardness and tenacity of subgingival calculus and the need for subsequent root planing. Local anaesthesia is often necessary, since pain may otherwise be experienced from sensitive root surfaces and the investing soft tissue. Instrumentation will be greatly facilitated by the chairside assistant providing a washed aspirated field.

The clinician should adopt a segmental approach, each tooth in the chosen segment being scaled and root planed to *completion* before moving to the next segment. This approach is preferable to the 'circuit' method where the entire mouth is part scaled at each appointment, increments of calculus being removed at each circuit until (hopefully!) none remains. The preferred, segmental method ensures maximal thoroughness and efficiency and it facilitates the use of local anaesthesia where necessary.

This latter approach, however, is not suitable for pockets which are sites of an intense inflammatory process since the scaling procedure may inadvertently extend beyond the base of the pocket, causing permanent loss of fibre attachment. In these cases, instrumentation should be a two-stage process; the initial subgingival scaling being carried out at a relatively superficial level, and without local anaesthetic so that pain responses are intact. The next scaling session should be postponed for about one month to allow for the establishment of new gingival collagen which will provide a landmark for the extension of further scaling and root planing.

The best results from subgingival débridement are often obtained from the combined use of hand and power-driven instruments to take advantage of their distinctive features and means of access to different parts of the pocket.

Hand instruments

'Scalers' is a generic term for the instruments used in scaling and root planing. These are produced by a large number of manufacturers, and instruments of the same type may vary greatly in size, shape and construction.

The head of a scaling instrument has a shank and a working tip (blade) of stainless steel or tungsten carbide. Although far more durable, some tungsten carbide blades are comparatively bulky, so that access to some pockets may be restricted.

Stainless steel blades become blunt quickly and must be sharpened frequently, sometimes during the course of a single treatment procedure. Tungsten carbide tips, being harder than steel, maintain their edge much longer.

A sharp scaler will 'grab' (engage) the root surface, and the surface layers of cementum will be removed by 'orthogonal' cutting along with attached plaque and calculus. A blunt scaler, on the other hand, slides over the root surface, burnishing it, without removing the irritant deposits. Heavy lateral pressure will be required to dislodge calculus with such an instrument, resulting in discomfort to the patient, as well as operator fatigue. The benefits of instrument sharpness cannot be overstated.

There are many different ways of sharpening scalers: for steel blades, the most acceptable technique involves the use of a handheld aluminium oxide stone (Arkansas stone). Tungsten carbide blades require a fine-grit diamond abrasive stone.

Scalers are classified as chisels, sickles, hoes and curettes (Fig. 10.1).

Push scaler (chisel scaler). This is used for removing calculus from proximal surfaces of mandibular anterior teeth. It is used from the labial aspect with a pen grasp and controlled push, with the fulcrum finger placed on the labial surfaces of adjacent teeth. It must be seated with extreme care to avoid gouging the root surface with one of the sharp corners.

Sickle scalers. These have two cutting edges on a straight or curved blade converging to a sharp point. They are used for supragingival scaling of proximal tooth surfaces. The cutting edge should be pulled coronally and, because there is an edge on both sides of the blade, they can be used on the distal aspect of one tooth and the mesial aspect of the adjacent tooth by the same basic approach with a slightly altered blade angle. Because of its design and size, the sickle scaler is not adaptable for subgingival use. Sickle scalers are available with curved shanks for use on posterior teeth.

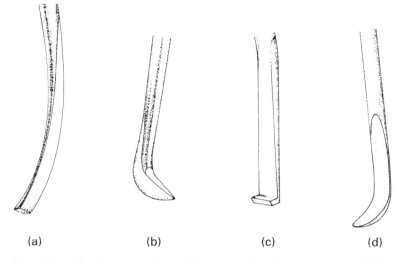

(a)   (b)   (c)   (d)

Fig. 10.1 Scalers: (a) chisel, (b) 'straight' sickle, (c) hoe and (d) curette.

Periodontal hoes. These have a cutting edge, set at right angles to the shank. A set of four different hoes is required to give access to all surfaces. Hoes are used to remove both supra- and subgingival calculus, although they are sometimes difficult to insert into pockets unless the marginal tissue is relatively flaccid. They are, however, invaluable for deep, narrow pockets which may not readily accommodate the full length of a curette blade. They are used with a coronally directed stroke and, like chisels, must be properly seated to avoid gouging the root surface.

Curettes. These instruments have a curved continuous spoon-shaped working end with one cutting edge (Gracey curettes) or two cutting edges (universal curettes). The back of the instrument is rounded. These instruments are unique amongst scalers in having no sharp corners or points which can gouge the root surface or lacerate the gingiva. The curette is, therefore, the instrument of choice for removing deep subgingival calculus and root planing.

Curettes are supplied in pairs. They vary in length, angulation and strength of shank, and in blade size and angulation. Long shanks are designed for posterior teeth and deep pockets; shanks with increased angulation are necessary for distal surfaces of posterior teeth; thick (rigid) shanks are better for heavy calculus deposits; large blades may be used when the tissue is loose and

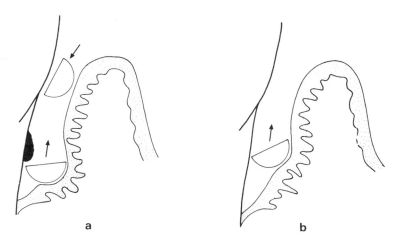

a   b

Fig. 10.2 Sectional diagrams showing a curette in use. (a) The blade is inserted subgingivally with the face flat against the tooth surface. To remove calculus, a working angulation of 80°–90° is adopted; (b) The root is planed with a reduced angulation of 50°–70°.

oedematous; and fine blades are necessary for subgingival instrumentation under firm fibrotic tissue. In use, curette blades should be aligned with the tooth surface as shown in Figure 10.2.

Power-driven scalers

Ultrasonic scalers

Magnetostrictive (electromagnetic) units. This is the traditional type of unit. It comprises a working tip, coupled to a stack of ferromagnetic metal in a high-frequency magnetic field. The 'stack' undergoes alternate expansion and contraction in response to application and removal of the magnetic field at a rate of about 25 000 cycles per second, and this results in a similar vibration frequency of the working tip. The amplitude of the vibratory movement is about 0.006–0.1 mm. The working tip describes an elliptical movement and, on contact with the tooth surface, adherent deposits are removed. Water flow through the tip dissipates heat and produces a cavitational effect, i.e. the water is atomized into tiny vacuum bubbles, and as they collapse the energy released helps to clear the field of plaque and loose debris.

Piezoelectric units. This is a second generation ultrasonic unit in which the magnetostriction stack is replaced by a quartz crystal mechanism. When an oscillating voltage is applied, the crystal system expands and contracts, resulting in high-frequency tip vibration which takes the form of a reciprocal, rather than elliptical motion. Less heat is produced and, therefore, less coolant is necessary, so reducing the need for aspiration.

Sonic (air-driven) scalers

Air-driven units work by compressed air activating a vibrating rod. These units are not ultrasonic but work at sonic frequencies (approximately 6000 cycles per second). They have the advantage of fitting readily into any dental unit with a compressed-air supply and, therefore, are relatively inexpensive. Sonic scalers, although more noisy and less powerful, appear to be as effective at removing calculus as ultrasonic scalers.

Use of power-driven scalers

When a power control is fitted to adjust the amplitude of tip movements, the lowest possible setting consistent with satisfactory resonance should be used to minimize trauma. With a pen grasp, the working tip is applied as parallel to the long axis of the tooth as possible. A light brushing type of stroke should be used with the minimum of pressure and the tip should be kept in motion at all times to avoid overheating any part of the tooth surface. It is essential to ensure that the water spray strikes the oscillating tip.

Indications

It has long been accepted that power-driven scalers can accomplish supragingival scaling at least as quickly as hand instruments. Furthermore, the cleansing effect of the water jet is a particular advantage when scaling a dirty mouth or one in which gingival bleeding is profuse. Patients usually experience less pain during ultrasonic instrumentation. This is a particularly important consideration in the treatment of acute necrotizing ulcerative gingivitis.

The use of power-driven scalers subgingivally has not met with as much general acceptance, since the clinician is unable to see the field, tactile sensation is poor and root surfaces cannot be planed. Nevertheless, there are numerous reports that power-driven scalers, compared with hand instrumentation, are equally effective in removing subgingival plaque and calculus, and the healing response to instrumentation is similar with both methods. Furthermore, since newly designed sonic and ultrasonic inserts allow greater access to the base of deep pockets and to furcations, it seems likely that power-driven scalers will increasingly be preferred to hand instruments.

Although power-driven scalers will remove contaminated cementum, some reports suggest that they create greater root surface roughness than hand curettes. This, however, is likely to be less important in the subgingival environment than supragingivally where the tooth surface is continuously exposed to plaque accumulation.

Power-driven scalers

Advantages	*Disadvantages*
Faster	Less tactile sensation
Less operator fatigue	Require water aspiration
Better patient acceptance	Produce contaminated aerosol
Less exacting technique	Less portable
Washed field visibility	Possible risk to pacemakers
No sharpening	Handpiece may be non-
Better access to furcations	autoclavable
Remove amalgam overhangs	

Pocket irrigation

After subgingival instrumentation, some clinicians irrigate pockets with a 0.2% solution of chlorhexidine. While there may be some slight benefit from the mechanical flushing effect, there is no clinical evidence of a significant chemical effect on the subgingival flora (see Chapter 16).

Healing after scaling and root planing

Healing processes: 1–2 weeks. Following subgingival instrumentation, bacterial remnants are washed out of the pocket by blood and gingival fluid. Within a few hours, an acute inflammatory reaction occurs in the soft-tissue pocket wall. Remnants of pocket epithelium proliferate and the pocket wall is fully epithelialized within 2 days. Involution of pocket epithelium gives rise to new junctional epithelium. After 5 days, epithelial reattachment commences at the apical extremity of the pocket, and progresses coronally until, under conditions of ideal plaque control, epithelial reattachment is complete in 14 days and a new gingival sulcus is formed near to the crest of the gingiva. At this time point, some gingival recession is apparent following reversal of the inflammatory swelling.

Healing processes: 3–6 weeks. The formation of functionally orientated collagen, to replace granulation tissue, does not commence until 3 weeks have elapsed. Probing depths continue to reduce until collagen regeneration is complete by which time resistance to probing is maximal. Most of the reduction in probing depth and gain in clinical attachment takes place within 6 weeks.

Healing processes: the later stages. Maturation of the connective tissue component may continue for several months. Where infrabony pockets have been treated, some bone-fill may occur, but perhaps not to the same extent as may be expected from surgical débridement, where a coagulum forms within the osseous defect.

Incomplete débridement. It is apparent that incomplete débridement may still be compatible with clinical periodontal health in many cases, and the necessary degree of root surface cleansing is likely to vary from patient to patient and from site to site. Success or failure of scaling and root planing may depend on a critical mass of plaque and calculus rather than its complete elimination.

Persistent disease. When healing fails to occur and inflammation persists, the cause may be attributed, either to further supragingival plaque accumulation followed by bacterial downgrowth, or to incomplete débridement with recolonization of the subgingival root surface from bacterial residues. Microbiological studies have shown that, following pocket débridement, if the tissues heal, few bacteria are recovered from the gingival sulcus. However, if insufficient pocket débridement has been performed, or supragingival plaque control has subsequently been inadequate, the original pocket microflora may be re-established in 4–6 weeks.

Instrumentation trauma. As subgingival débridement is carried out, a certain amount of instrumentation trauma occurs, leading to minor amounts of attachment loss. This is certainly apparent for initially shallow pockets (up to 3 mm deep before treatment). However, the resistance to probing produced by repair processes in deeper pockets (initially 4–6 mm deep) is thought to mask any loss of connective tissue attachment which may occur at these sites. Indeed, in pockets of more than 6 mm initial probing depth, so great is the resistance to probing after treatment that, in spite of any damage which the fibre attachment at the base of the pocket might sustain, improved clinical attachment levels are usually recorded on probing.

Periodontal surgery

'Periodontal surgery' is a term normally reserved for procedures requiring the use of a scalpel. Surgical procedures in current use include:

Surgical procedures
1. Gingivectomy to remove excess gingival tissue.
2. Flap procedures to improve access to the root surface for completion of root instrumentation in cases of advanced periodontitis.
3. Root separation and resection where periodontitis involves the furcation regions of multirooted teeth.
4. Mucogingival surgery for gingival augmentation and root coverage.
5. Surgical crown lengthening incorporating gingivectomy or flap procedures.
6. Regenerative techniques which seek to renew the connective tissue attachment apparatus.

For convenience, root separation and resection are described in Chapter 13, mucogingival surgery in Chapter 17, surgical crown lengthening in Chapter 21 and periodontal regeneration in Chapter 12. Only the gingivectomy procedure and flap surgery for periodontitis are discussed here. The reader's attention is drawn to the descriptions of structural changes during healing and the rationale of surgical treatment considered in Chapter 7.

The gingivectomy procedure

Indications

Fibrous gingival overgrowth. Mild gingival overgrowth is common in simple gingivitis, particularly around crowded teeth or within relief areas of partial dentures. In its most severe form it is associated with systemic modifying factors (see Chapter 3). Surgical removal of the enlarged tissues may be desirable: for

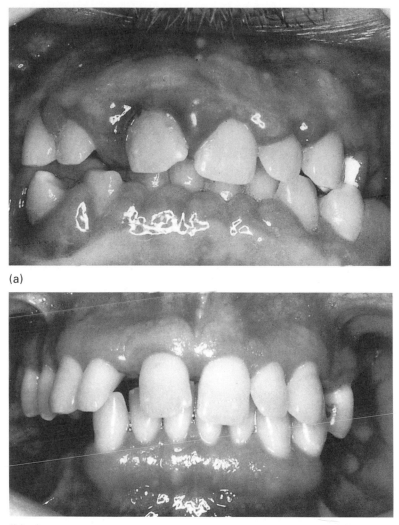

(a)

(b)

Fig. 11.1 Hereditary gingival fibromatosis: (a) before gingivectomy; (b) after gingivectomy.

cosmetic reasons; because of interference with occlusion; to facilitate operative dental surgery or prosthodontic work; in combination with a flap procedure for underlying periodontitis; or because the bulky gingiva appears to prevent adequate oral hygiene (Fig. 11.1).

Subgingival restoration margins. Restorations located below the gingival margin tend to promote subgingival plaque accumulation. Gingivectomy may result in a permanently located supragingival margin or may simply provide temporary access to insert a new restoration with a better marginal finish (see Chapter 21).

Epulides. These localized polypoidal gingival lesions (see Chapter 5) may be sessile or pedunculated. Although a gingivectomy incision may be used to remove the bulk of the lesion, it is essential afterwards to excise the base of the lesion down to bone, and to remove tooth surface irritants thoroughly. Histological examination of the excised tissue is mandatory.

Importance of plaque control. In patients predisposed to gingival overgrowth, inadequate plaque control after surgery will result in recurrent enlargement. Therefore, patient commitment and manual dexterity must be tested during a presurgical phase of hygiene therapy. In patients with persistently poor plaque control in spite of oral hygiene instruction, the clinician may decide that the problem is not sufficiently severe to justify the short-term advantage of gingivectomy. On the other hand, a good response to hygiene therapy may result in tissue shrinkage sufficient to obviate the need for surgery. Very occasionally, gingival overgrowth is so severe that it is unreasonable to expect the patient to achieve good supragingival plaque control, and surgery may proceed without the patient reaching the oral hygiene level normally expected prior to surgical intervention in the hope that better standards of home care can be achieved afterwards.

Technique

Following anaesthesia, a bevelled incision through the gingiva is directed at the base of the pocket (Fig. 11.2). The detached gingiva is removed and the exposed tooth surface instrumented. To protect the wound, a periodontal dressing is adapted to the wound surface and left in place for one week.

In the surgical treatment of gross gingival overgrowth, an open-wound gingivectomy may be combined with an undermining flap operation to avoid the creation of a large connective tissue wound.

Healing after gingivectomy

From the second postoperative day onwards, epithelial cells migrate over the wound surface from the wound margin

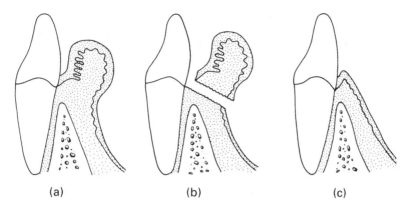

(a)   (b)   (c)

Fig. 11.2 Gingivectomy. (a) Fibrous gingival enlargement; (b)
bevelled incision; (c) formation of new marginal gingiva.

towards the tooth at the rate of about 0.5 mm per day. Epithelialization, therefore, is barely complete by the time of dressing
removal, and keratinization takes a further 2 weeks. Proliferation of fibroblasts adjacent to the wound surface occurs, leading
to coronal regrowth of tissue and the formation of a new free
gingival unit by about the seventh postoperative day. The
formation and maturation of collagen takes place from about
the third week as a new epithelial attachment is formed.
Complete healing of the gingivectomy wound takes about 6
weeks but minor dimensional changes may continue for several
months.

Surgical treatment of periodontitis

Aims

The principal aim of surgical intervention in the treatment of
periodontitis is the provision of good access for the completion
of scaling and root planing, thereby creating a physiological
gingival sulcus and preserving connective tissue attachment.

Unlike hyperplastic gingivitis, periodontitis is a disease
usually with very limited effect on gingival contour and on the
access to *visible* tooth surfaces for self-performed plaque control.
Surgery is not, therefore, performed in order to *create* good gingival contours. However, it is important to employ a technique of
surgery which will allow the *re-establishment* of favourable gingival contours during healing.

Objectives

The ultimate objective of periodontal therapy must be the regeneration of predisease quantities of healthy periodontium. However, at present, there are practical difficulties in achieving this (see Chapter 12). We are usually obliged to accept as a realistic objective the restoration to health of remaining periodontal support, i.e. the arrest, but not reversal, of connective tissue attachment loss.

Indications

Surgery is indicated after a phase of hygiene therapy for residual deep pathological (bleeding) pockets at sites where plaque control is good.

Significance of probing depth. Careful reference to the treatment planning chart is necessary. If hygiene therapy has been properly carried out and good oral hygiene has been established, there will be no *shallow* pathological pockets since these will have been instrumented adequately. Residual pathological pockets will be those where access for non-surgical instrumentation was poor and these pockets will be relatively deep.

Assessment of plaque control. It is not sufficient that oral hygiene is *generally* good. If the patient cannot clean the *sites* being considered for surgery, treatment will fail. An exception may, however, be made for patients who find flossing difficult if sufficient interdental space is expected to develop postoperatively to accommodate an interdental brush. Where doubt exists concerning the adequacy of plaque control, surgery may be carried out for a single segment of the dentition and further surgery postponed until the adequacy of postoperative plaque control can be confirmed.

Choice of technique

Surgical techniques for the treatment of periodontitis are sometimes differentiated by the priority given to pocket elimination or reattachment. The main differences are in the management of bone and method of wound closure; the main objective in each case is a physiological gingival sulcus. During 'pocket elimination', the soft tissue forming the pocket wall is resected or repositioned apically with formation, during healing, of a new gingival margin at a more apical level. Bony pocket walls are also resected. 'Reattachment' requires the preservation of gingival soft tissue with formation of a long epithelial attachment to the planed root surface. Often elements of both reattachment and pocket elimination are combined in one procedure.

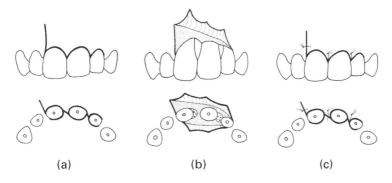

(a)   (b)   (c)

Fig. 11.3 Open-flap curettage. (a) Marginal intracrevicular and vertical relieving incisions; (b) buccal and palatal mucoperiosteal flaps reflected to expose marginal bone and interdental bone defects; (c) wound closure with simple interrupted sutures.

It is of fundamental importance that details of surgical technique are not allowed to obscure the prerequisites for successful surgery, namely adequate débridement at operation and adequate plaque control subsequently.

In this text, the technique mostly recommended is 'open-flap curettage', a reattachment procedure. Pocket elimination is also described as an alternative approach which is mainly applicable around molars.

Open-flap curettage

Flaps are elevated with minimal sacrifice of soft tissue to give access for root instrumentation, then replaced at or close to their presurgical position, eventually to form an epithelial attachment to the cleaned tooth surface.

1. A marginal incision is made within the pocket or gingival sulcus around the necks of teeth buccally, lingually and proximally (Fig. 11.3(a)).
2. If a deep pocket is present at one end of the marginal incision, a vertical relieving incision may be required on the buccal aspect to provide proper access. Vertical incisions are unnecessary on lingual or palatal aspects.
3. Full-thickness mucoperiosteal flaps are elevated on both buccal and lingual/palatal aspects to expose the marginal bone (Fig. 11.3(b)).
4. Granulation tissue adhering to the bone is removed and the roots are scaled and planed until hard and smooth.

5. Bone contouring may occasionally be necessary to reduce sharp edges or facilitate flap closure. Bone contours, however, should not be adjusted purely to make them conform to some imagined 'physiological' ideal. This could result in loss of support to adjacent unaffected tooth surfaces. In any case, many defects, particularly those with three walls, possess good potential for bone-fill.

6. The flaps are replaced with interrupted sutures (Fig. 11.3(c)). Periodontal dressing is unnecessary since complete wound closure should have been achieved.

7. Sutures are removed one week later.

Healing after open-flap curettage

When close adaptation of buccal and lingual flap margins is achieved following open-flap curettage, healing by primary intention may occur. Sometimes, however, the tissue contraction associated with wound healing prevents the union of buccal and lingual flap margins and a soft-tissue interdental crater is produced. Most craters resolve spontaneously within 6 months, but careful attention must be paid to interdental plaque control during this time.

The pocket epithelium, which has been replaced against the root surface, undergoes involution and forms junctional epithelium. A mature epithelial attachment forms in 2–4 weeks. When intrabony lesions are present, bone-fill may occur within the boundaries of the bone defect, usually accompanied by some crestal resorption. There will, however, be a strand of junctional epithelium interposed between the regenerated bone tissue and the root surface.

Advantages of open-flap curettage

1. Rapid healing is achieved with minimal postoperative discomfort, and periodontal dressing is usually unnecessary.

2. With no exposed areas to granulate and epithelialize, patients are soon able to resume mechanical plaque control instead of relying on chlorhexidine for a lengthy period with its inconvenient side-effects.

3. The repair potential of tissues affected by periodontitis is fully exploited, periodontal support preserved, and increased tooth mobility avoided.

4. Postoperative recession is minimized (Fig. 11.4), giving optimum aesthetics, minimal exposure of sensitive dentine and minimal risk of root caries and speech impairment.

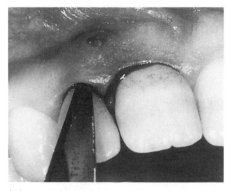

Fig. 11.4 Severe periodontitis affecting 12. (a) By making an intracrevicular incision, and (b) retaining all the supporting bone, recession (c) is minimized.

(a)

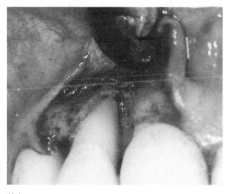

(b)

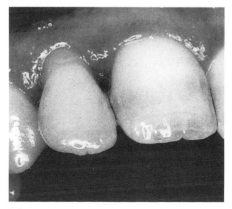

(c)

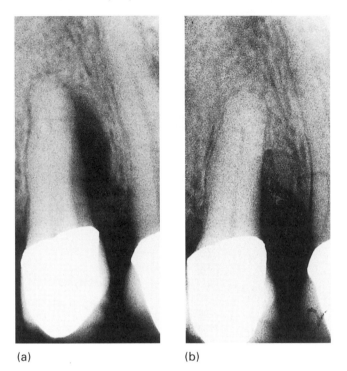

(a)   (b)

Fig. 11.5 Bone-fill after open-flap curettage: (a)
before surgery; (b) after surgery.

5. Supporting bone can be retained and optimal bone-fill
    within angular defects should be achieved (Fig. 11.5).
6. Longitudinal studies have shown that, in the treatment of
    deep pockets, this technique leads to a greater gain of clini-
    cal attachment than that obtainable by any other surgical
    method in routine use.

Pocket elimination

Using the technique outlined above in molar regions, flaps which
are replaced close to their presurgical position may collapse into
wide proximal bone defects, leading to a protracted remodelling
process, during which plaque control will be impaired. To avoid
this, the surgical technique may be modified to achieve a more
harmonious gingival contour early in the healing process. Thus,
it may be advisable, with as little destruction of supporting bone
as possible, to reduce the depth of bone defects (Fig. 11.6(a)), to

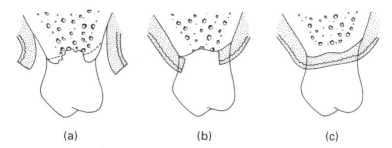

(a)　　　　　　(b)　　　　　　(c)

Fig. 11.6 Pocket elimination for molar periodontitis. (a) Buccal and palatal flaps reflected; broken line indicates extent of planned osteoplasty. (b) Flaps replaced after osteoplasty. (c) Interdental gingival contour after healing of exposed interdental bone.

trim and/or apically position the flaps and to secure them at the level of the newly contoured bone crest (Fig. 11.6(b)). Soft tissue coverage of interdental bone is usually incomplete and a periodontal dressing may be required, both to protect the wound and help to adapt the soft tissue to the crestal bone.

This pocket elimination approach will create a new marginal gingiva and dentogingival junction of normal dimensions at a more apical level, close to the base of the original pocket (Fig. 11.6(c)). Although gingival recession is produced, aesthetic considerations are less important in molar segments. Indeed the gingival recession may be beneficial: since much of the affected root surface will not be covered by soft tissue, any irritant root deposits, still present after surgical débridement, are less likely to provoke inflammation; and in the event of recurrent periodontitis, the pathological pockets which form should be shallow and easy to instrument.

Other indications for surgical pocket elimination include subgingival caries and restoration margins.

Planning of periodontal surgery

All teeth must be accessible both for surgery and subsequent home care. Upper second and third molars may be particularly awkward because of the proximity of the coronoid process of the mandible when the mouth is open. There may be a small oral aperture, narrow arches or a hyperactive tongue as well as peculiarities of tooth position.

Surgery may be carried out in sextants, quadrants, arches, half or whole mouths according to circumstances. Complex techniques, such as those which may be required to manage furcation lesions, should generally be restricted to one sextant. Although the patient may be less inconvenienced by a surgical programme condensed into one or two extended appointments, it is the clinician's responsibility to ensure that too much is not attempted at one sitting, so that the procedure may be completed satisfactorily without leaving clinician or patient physically or emotionally drained. The tolerance of the patient and finesse of the operator may be stretched if periodontal surgical procedures are extended beyond 45–60 minutes.

Surgical principles

Local anaesthesia should commence whenever possible by block injection to minimize the number of injections. Teeth, as well as periodontium, should be anaesthetized to avoid eliciting pain during scaling and root planing. When anaesthesia has been achieved, papillary infiltration is employed to reduce blood loss and improve visibility.

Management of soft tissue. Following initial incisions for flap procedures, full-thickness (mucoperiosteal) flaps are raised by blunt dissection. The flap should be elevated only as far as is necessary to gain access or achieve any desired repositioning. Gauze sponges moistened with saline may be used at various stages during surgery to contain haemorrhage within interdental spaces. Removal of granulation tissue will further reduce haemorrhage and facilitate inspection of bone margins and root furcations. It is often only at this stage that final decisions can be taken about bone recontouring and flap closure.

Management of bone. When bone removal is necessary, recontouring should be carried out as atraumatically as possible using appropriately shaped burs or coarse-bonded diamond stones rotating slowly with adequate saline irrigation, or using hand-held chisels or files.

Management of tooth substance. The recontouring of tooth substance is undertaken most frequently in relation to early furcation involvement and this will be dealt with in Chapter 13. However, on occasion, it will be desirable to reduce the groove sometimes found on the palatal aspect of upper incisors or the root furrows of posterior teeth, notably upper first premolars. This should be carried out judiciously, bearing in mind the risk of postoperative dentine sensitivity and caries.

Postoperative sequelae

These should be anticipated and patients warned in advance. In common with other forms of oral surgery, postoperative pain and swelling may occur but will usually be mild and transient. Acute or pyogenic wound infection is rare. Postoperative bleeding is usually easily controlled if the bleeding area is identified and pressure applied.

Hypermobility. Tooth mobility frequently increases after periodontal surgery and may not peak until 3 weeks later. It will then decline over 3–6 months to preoperative levels or less, provided supporting bone has not been removed. Teeth associated with angular bone defects, and mobile before surgery, may be stabilized if bone-fill occurs.

Dentine hypersensitivity. Large areas of newly planed root surface may be exposed to chemical, thermal and mechanical stimuli. This may be severe enough to preclude adequate tooth cleaning and may reflect a transient pulpal hyperaemia due to the instrumentation of the root surface. Loss of the insulating layer of gingival soft tissue will make the patient more aware of thermal stimuli. Dentine hypersensitivity should be treated aggressively with fluoride preparations so that plaque is not left to accumulate in sensitive areas and cause recurrent periodontal disease.

Postoperative care

It is of fundamental importance that operated tooth surfaces do not become plaque-infected during healing or indeed subsequently. To this end, patients must be given detailed instruction in the home care of operated and adjacent areas in the postoperative period and be seen frequently enough to ensure that the instructions are carried out and that they are effective. Mechanical cleaning in the operated area will be limited in scope for the first 2 weeks after surgery. Chlorhexidine mouthwash is prescribed so that the patient will be spared the discomfort of cleaning tender gingivae and sensitive root surfaces. This regimen should be continued until cleaning can take place mechanically without bleeding or discomfort.

When, in spite of efforts to avoid it at the time of surgery, a soft-tissue crater develops postoperatively, the use of chlorhexidine may have to be continued for a few weeks. With meticulous plaque control, gingiva will tend to seek a scalloped contour which will facilitate subsequent mechanical plaque control measures. If plaque infection of root surfaces is allowed to occur, either epithelial attachment will not take place and a pocket will result, or gingival regeneration will be suppressed.

With the reinstitution of mechanical cleaning, oral hygiene measures should be reappraised in light of the gingival recession which has taken place. Interdental spaces will be larger and a correspondingly larger interdental brush may be required. Patients with no preoperative interdental space may be able to use an interdental brush after surgery. Patients should be made aware that relatively rough root surfaces, newly exposed, will take longer to clean than smooth enamel. Proximal root concavities may accumulate supragingival plaque for the first time and will require special attention.

Satisfactory results will be achieved and untoward sequelae avoided only if a regimen of close supervision for reinforcement of oral hygiene is adopted. Patients should be seen frequently until the clinician is satisfied that adequate oral hygiene is being maintained, when the interval between recall visits may be gradually extended (see Chapter 19).

Periodontal regeneration

In routine clinical practice, a realistic aim for the treatment of periodontitis is the restoration to health of remaining periodontal support, i.e. the arrest but not reversal of connective tissue attachment loss. Thus, during healing, epithelial reattachment to the previously diseased root surface occurs. However, the ideal goal of periodontal therapy is the regeneration of predisease quantities of healthy supporting tissue comprising new alveolar bone, periodontal ligament and cementum, forming a new connective tissue attachment.

Substantial research work suggests that wound healing with the formation of a new connective tissue attachment is a process of great complexity involving proliferation and migration of periodontal ligament cells, synthesis of extracellular matrix and differentiation of cementoblasts and osteoblasts. A variety of methods has been employed to facilitate the regenerative process, and these are summarized below.

Bone replacement grafts

Early attempts at regenerative surgery involved various types of graft material, packed into angular bone defects and covered with soft tissue. These materials are thought to possess at least one of the following properties:

Bone replacement grafts should be:
- Osteogenic: able to form new bone through the activity of graft cells.
- Osteoconductive: able to serve as a scaffold for adjacent host bone.
- Osteoinductive: able to stimulate bone growth within adjacent soft tissue.

The list of materials tested now includes: fresh autogenous bone and marrow from the iliac crest or from intra-oral sites; frozen, autogenous or allogenic cancellous bone and marrow from the iliac crest; demineralized or non-demineralized, freeze-dried, allogenic cortical bone; biodegradable synthetic graft materials including tricalcium phosphate and natural coral (calcium carbonate); and non-absorbable synthetic materials such as hydroxyapatite and bioactive glass. Several studies have observed little or no advantage to osseous grafting over non-grafted controls with respect to the amount of bone-fill achieved, and epithelialization of the root-surface–graft-tissue interface is a frequent outcome. While there is limited evidence that some new connective tissue attachment occurs after the use of autogenous bone and marrow, especially from the iliac crest, root resorption and ankylosis is a common side-effect unless the graft material has been frozen. Demineralized freeze-dried bone allograft has been shown to facilitate new connective tissue attachment but cannot be wholeheartedly recommended because of the risk of disease transmission, however slight. Synthetic materials function primarily as biocompatible space fillers leading to significant improvements in probing depths and clinical attachment levels, but not giving rise to periodontal regeneration.

Root surfacing conditioning

Citric acid conditioning of surgically exposed root surfaces has been shown to dissolve the smear layer formed by root planing, to detoxify remaining root surface contaminant, and to demineralize the dentine surface, exposing collagen fibrils of the dentine matrix. These exposed fibrils are thought to improve the adhesion, proliferation and migration of fibroblasts on the root surface and to interdigitate with newly formed collagen fibrils in the healing tissue. Thus, citric acid conditioning ought to facilitate early adhesion of the fibrin coagulum to the root surface, thereby preventing apical migration of epithelial cells, as well as setting in motion the desired maturation and organization of granulation tissue. The effect of citric acid has been tested in experimental animals with conflicting results and in humans generally with little success.

Surgical technique

Whatever regenerative technique is employed, a traditional reverse-bevel incision, rather than an intracrevicular incision, must be used so that when the flap is readapted to the root surface it will be virtually devoid of epithelium on its inner surface. Furthermore, a technique should be employed which will leave the root-surface–coagulum interface protected from mechanical injury during healing. In this respect, improvement in the healing of furcation defects has been achieved with wound closure techniques which stabilize the flap in a more coronal location, where movement of its margin has little impact on the critical healing area. Failure to accomplish postoperative flap stability may encourage epithelial colonization of the root surface. The difficulties in obtaining adequate wound protection may explain why success with citric acid root conditioning is frequently not achieved.

Guided tissue regeneration

There is considerable evidence that only cells originating from the periodontal ligament are capable of producing a connective tissue attachment and that, if the root becomes populated instead by gingival connective tissue cells or bone cells, resorption of its surface may occur. Preferential colonization of root surfaces by cells from the periodontal ligament can be achieved by a process known as guided tissue regeneration (GTR). This involves the placement of a porous membrane (barrier) underneath the surgical flap, extending from the *outer* surface of the alveolar process to the crown of the tooth just apical to the gingival margin (Fig. 12.1).

Membrane barriers

The first commercially available barrier was manufactured from expanded polytetrafluoroethylene or 'ePTFE' (Gore-tex Periodontal Material®). The coronal border of this membrane has an open microstructure allowing ingrowth of connective tissue to prevent apical migration of epithelium down the outside of the barrier. The remainder of the membrane is occlusive, preventing the gingival tissues outside the membrane from interfering with the healing process at the root surface (Fig. 12.1). This allows periodontal ligament cells to populate the root surface, although, theoretically, bone cells could also have access to the root. Follow-up surgery is necessary to remove the membrane.

In recent years, equivalent results have been obtained using bioabsorbable membranes of polylactic and polyglycolic acid.

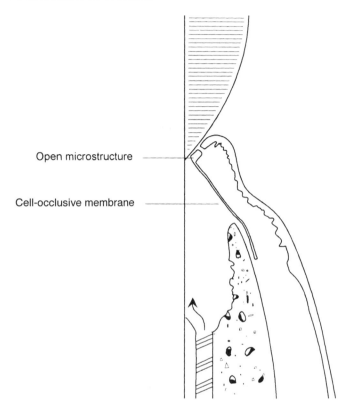

Open microstructure

Cell-occlusive membrane

Fig. 12.1 Guided tissue regeneration, depicting Gore-tex Periodontal Material® *in situ* following surgical débridement of an infrabony pocket.

Use of these materials eliminates the need for follow-up surgery to remove the barrier.

Case selection

Guided tissue regeneration is advocated mainly for deep multiwall bone defects and grade II furcation lesions. It should be possible for a clot to form within these defects without being displaced by the membrane, allowing colonization of the root surface by periodontal ligament cells. It is, of course, essential that the root surface is fully accessible to scaling instruments. Guided tissue regeneration is not a substitute for thorough débridement.

Barrier membranes, in conjunction with pedicle graft procedures, can also be used to treat deep recession defects provided a space for tissue formation can be created under the membrane (see Chapter 17).

Stringent criteria must be applied in selecting suitable lesions for treatment and, even then, regeneration is frequently incomplete. It should be noted that the lesions for which GTR techniques are currently designed – moderately deep angular bone defects – are also those which respond favourably to conventional open flap curettage by bony repair. GTR surgery should be used to obtain enhanced attachment levels at these sites, and should never be used as a last ditch attempt to save teeth which have so little fibre attachment remaining that they can no longer provide a rich source of periodontal ligament progenitor cells.

Membrane barriers are expensive and cost-benefit factors must inevitably be a major consideration in case selection.

Clinical outcomes

Using GTR techniques in the treatment of deep infrabony pockets, it has been shown that, compared to conventional open flap curettage, more clinical attachment gain occurs (on average, 3.5 mm v 2.00 mm) with less residual probing depth (on average, 3.00 mm v 4.00 mm).

With regard to furcation defects, mandibular lesions with angular bone loss have emerged as the ones most likely to benefit from GTR techniques. However, these benefits are relatively modest and unpredictable. Horizontal clinical attachment gain amounts, on average, to only 2.5 mm v 1.5 mm from open flap curettage, with complete closure in less than 50% of cases.

In spite of careful adherence to the proper surgical technique, there is a tendency for gingival recession to occur, exposing the coronal portion of the membrane with subsequent bacterial contamination which may affect adversely the regenerative capacity of the tissues. The surgical trauma caused by removal of non-resorbable membranes may further prejudice the regenerative process.

Those factors which spoil the outcome of conventional surgery are equally detrimental to GTR surgery. Thus, smoking or failure to maintain adequate plaque control at GTR-treated sites are likely to result in recurrent disease.

The future

Current regenerative procedures are technically demanding and unpredictable, and many other avenues of research are being explored. For instance, it has been shown that enamel matrix proteins, which are deposited on root surfaces during embryogenesis, promote the subsequent formation of cementum, periodontal ligament and alveolar bone. Clinical trials of porcine enamel matrix derivative in the form of a commercially available gel (Emdogain®), which is applied to surgically exposed and citric acid-etched root surfaces, have already been undertaken, so far demonstrating modest improvements in clinical attachment levels.

Management of furcation lesions

A furcation lesion ('furcation involvement') is an extension of periodontitis between the roots of multirooted teeth, typically the molars and upper first premolars. The only peculiarity of the lesion is its anatomical situation. In all other respects the lesion is similar to that on a single-rooted tooth. It is the inaccessibility of the lesion which necessitates special mention. Pulp pathology may also give rise to furcation lesions and is discussed in Chapter 14.

Classification

There is wide acceptance of three stages of furcation lesion, but no consensus on the grading criteria. The following classification is used in this text.

Classification of furcation lesions
Grade I – incipient, up to 3 mm of *horizontal* attachment loss.
Grade II – between incipient and through-and-through.
Grade III – through-and-through involvement.

Aetiology

Although the primary aetiological factor is bacterial plaque, variation in tooth morphology has a major influence on the frequency with which different furcation sites are affected and on the ensuing pattern of destruction.

Cervical enamel projections are common at molar furcation sites and are associated with an increased risk of furcation disease.

Approximately 50% of upper first premolars have two roots. The majority of upper first molars have three roots and most lower first molars have two. Second and third molars are less predictable and exhibit more variations on this basic pattern. Length, curvature and divergence of roots vary widely, as does the length of root trunk (the distance between the amelocemental junction and the furcation). This distance may be different for each furcation of the same tooth and, indeed, any individual furcation may be absent because of fusion of adjacent roots. Roots which are distinctly separate coronally may be fused apically.

Occurrence and distribution

Furcation disease is extremely common among patients with periodontitis. Upper molars are affected slightly more frequently than lower molars. In either jaw, second molars are affected almost as often as first molars and much more frequently than third molars. Furcation disease affects buccal sites in both jaws and lower lingual sites with a similar frequency but is most prevalent at distal sites of upper first molars. These facts can be explained largely by length of root trunk and accessibility for plaque control.

Diagnosis

A sound knowledge of root anatomy is invaluable to the clinician dealing with furcation lesions. The upper first molar (Fig. 13.1), for example, has a mesiobuccal root, often narrow mesiodistally (as seen on radiograph), but normally broad buccopalatally. The palatal root tends to be thick, straight and round in cross-section, but frequently diverges from the long axis of the tooth and may be affected by recession. It tends to be situated distally. Thus, the mesial furcation will be more readily examined from the palatal aspect (Fig. 13.2). The distal root is usually the smallest in cross-section and length. The distal furcation tends to be displaced slightly in a buccal direction owing to the greater diameter of the palatal root, and so the distal furcation is usually examined from the buccal side. Because of the small circumference of the distobuccal root, grade III furcation involvement is likely to occur first between the buccal and distal furcations.

Furcation lesions can be diagnosed by careful clinical examination, ideally using a curved periodontal probe. It should be possible to feel the roof of the furcation in this way, so confirming its involvement. Radiographic examination, possibly using

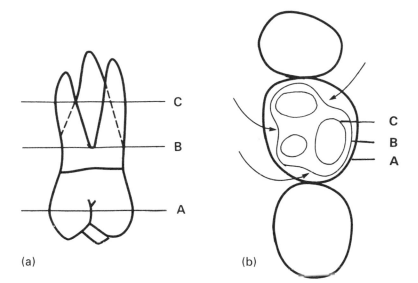

Fig. 13.1 The upper molar trifurcation. (a) Upper first molar seen from the buccal aspect showing three planes of section A, B, C. (b) Cross-section through upper first molar showing levels A, B, C (superimposed). Level A illustrates the relationship of the crown to adjacent teeth. Level B shows the entrances to the trifurcation (arrowed). Level C indicates the relative size and position of the three roots.

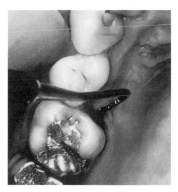

Fig. 13.2 Williams periodontal probe in the mesial furcation of an upper first molar. Note how far palatally the furcation is situated owing to the breadth of the mesiobuccal root.

the parallax technique, may reveal additional detail. However, because of the superimposition of roots in the upper premolar and molar areas, the extent of involvement can easily be under-estimated, and so radiographs should not be relied upon. The full extent of furcation involvement may be difficult to evaluate without resort to surgical exploration.

Treatment options

The treatment procedures about to be described apply mainly to molar furcation lesions: upper first premolars are rarely responsive to any form of treatment once furcation disease is established, because the furcation entrances are located on the proximal surfaces, usually in the mid-third of the root, and the separate roots are usually too small and slender for root resection to be contemplated.

Treatment options
1. Scaling and root planing.
2. Open-flap curettage.
3. Apically repositioned flap.
4. Guided tissue regeneration.
5. Tunnel preparation.
6. Root resection.
7. Palliative care/extraction.

Scaling and root planing

The aim of conventional débridement is to eliminate the inflammatory lesion and effect repair of the damaged periodontium with epithelial reattachment. Scaling and root planing without surgical access is likely to be wholly effective only for some grade I lesions. Furcation openings are often narrower than the width of a curette and there are plaque retentive concavities within. Even if full access is possible with curettes or hoes, space to manipulate the instrument within the furcation is often limited. Ultrasonic scalers may, therefore, be more effective than hand scalers.

Open-flap curettage

By obtaining surgical access, scaling and root planing may be extended to treatment of grade II lesions, although success is unpredictable especially at buccal or lingual sites. Failure can be attributed either to incomplete removal of furcation plaque or postoperative breakdown of the fibrin clot within the defect and ingress of bacteria during the early healing phase. Access for completion of scaling and root planing may, if necessary, be obtained by reshaping the furcation entrance, but this should be done cautiously to avoid pulp complications. Tapered cylindrical rotary instruments coated with fine diamond particles ('root diamonds') may be used both to carry out the 'furcation-plasty' and to help débride the furcation. When closing the wound, the furcation entrance should be covered with the flap, using, if necessary, a periosteal relieving incision to advance the flap coronally.

Apically repositioned flap procedure

This procedure is similar to open-flap curettage, except that the flap is sutured *apical* to the furcation entrance leaving the furcation bone to granulate over, so that as healing proceeds the furcation becomes partially filled with gingival tissue. This approach should be reserved for highly motivated patients whose plaque control skills are sufficiently developed to clean thoroughly *within* the exposed furcation entrance.

Guided tissue regeneration

The ideal outcome of treatment is the regeneration of lost supporting tissue including the formation of a new connective tissue attachment. In carefully selected cases this is wholly or partially achievable by 'guided tissue regeneration' (GTR) (see Fig. 13.3 overleaf), the principles of which are discussed in Chapter 12. Comparative studies have shown that GTR procedures with barrier membranes may result in significant clinical improvement beyond that achieved by open débridement alone in grade I or small grade II buccal or lingual furcation lesions. Mandibular lesions are more predictable than maxillary lesions.

Proximal furcation lesions and molars with gingival recession or with short root trunks, large furcation defects, or furcation defects that cannot be adequately scaled are unsuitable for guided tissue regeneration, and outcomes are significantly impaired by tobacco smoking and inadequate postoperative plaque control.

Tunnel preparation

Deep grade II and grade III lesions are unlikely to respond to open flap curettage with or without the placement of a barrier membrane. In these cases the loss of furcation tissue integrity should be regarded as permanent, and a tunnel procedure consid-

a)   b)   c)   d)

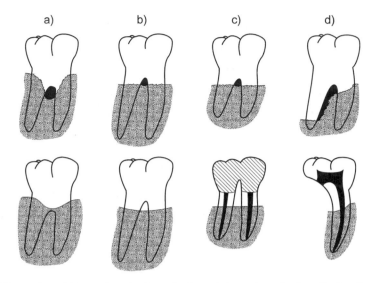

Fig. 13.3 Bifurcation lesions before (above) and after (below) treatment by: (a) guided tissue regeneration; note the long root trunk and good proximal bone support; (b) tunnel preparation with bone removal; note the short root trunk and proximal bone loss; (c) tunnel preparation without bone removal, incorporating root separation and linked crowns; note the short roots; (d) root resection; note the unequal bone support.

ered. This involves making the furcation accessible to daily plaque control and is most often applicable to lower molars with a short root trunk and long, widely separated roots (see Fig. 13.3). After buccal and lingual flaps are elevated, sufficient interradicular bone must be removed with a bur to accommodate the healing gingiva and leave a patent tunnel through which an interdental brush can be passed. Tunnel procedures can also be performed for upper molars in conjunction with resection of one root, usually the disto-buccal root. Although good initial results may be obtained by tunnel procedures, there is a significant risk of caries especially within the plaque-retentive irregularities of mandibular molar furcations, exposed for the first time to dietary carbohydrate.

Where removal of interradicular bone is undesirable, the roots can be separated completely after first performing endodontic treatment, and a higher roof provided for the furcation by means of a 'double crown' (see Fig. 13.3). This eliminates the risk of caries within the furcation dome but leaves the tooth exposed to the risk of endodontic treatment failure.

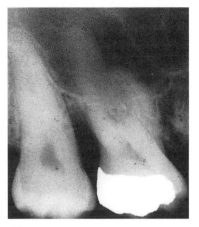

(a)

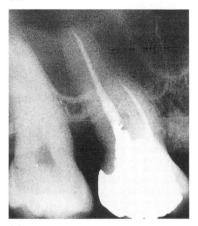

(b)

Fig. 13.4 Root resection: (a) distal furcation lesion affecting 16; (b) crown contour after removal of the distobuccal root; (c) radiographic appearance one year later.

(c)

Root resection

Many grade II or III furcation lesions are inaccessible for scaling and root planing even with surgical access, and are also unsuitable for tunnel procedures. Their certain elimination can be achieved only by root resection (Figs 13.3 and 13.4). This is a much more invasive approach to the problem of furcation disease since root canal therapy is necessary, and crown or bridge preparation is often required afterwards. Not surprisingly, the majority of failures associated with root resection are of endodontic origin or attributable to root fracture, rather than recurrent periodontitis, the risk of which is lower than with other furcation treatment modalities. A decision to proceed with root resection is often made when conservative treatment has failed. The following factors should be considered.

Root selection. The choice of root(s) to be retained will be dictated by location of the furcation lesion, amount of residual bone supporting the individual roots, their strategic position within the arch and the feasibility of root canal therapy.

Endodontics. It is desirable, but not essential, that the roots to be retained are endodontically treated before separation. Sometimes, however, a definite decision about which root or roots to retain can be made only after surgical exploration or division of the crown and roots, to allow assessment of mobility and probing of the furcation surfaces of the roots. In such circumstances of doubtful prognosis, endodontic treatment may be delayed until after surgery. It is essential to retain sufficient tooth substance to facilitate application of rubber dam and subsequent restoration of the tooth.

Surgical technique. Buccal and lingual flaps should always be raised, and the process of sectioning should start in the affected furcation. The cut should be made with a sharp bur or diamond stone, and should be wide enough to allow space for elevation of the root to be removed. Care should be taken not to leave behind part of the roof of the furcation, a common mistake if access is not created by flap elevation.

Mobility and occlusion. The mobility of individual roots after separation may exceed the mobility of the whole tooth, and the remaining portion of tooth should be relieved of eccentric occlusal contact if it appears very mobile after surgery. Some reduction of mobility can be expected as healing proceeds.

Restoration. Sometimes, the coronal portion of the tooth may be relatively intact following root resection (see Fig. 13.4). In other cases, artificial crown construction is necessary. The tooth morphology achieved by root resection is often less than ideal: the furcation aspect of the remaining root(s), to which any subsequent restoration must conform, is frequently concave and plaque retentive; and the restoration margin, which must extend beyond the floor of the pulp chamber, may have to be located subgingivally close to the alveolar crest, unless sufficient bone loss has already occurred or bone removal is undertaken.

Palliative care/extraction

Teeth with grade II or III involvement which are not to receive definitive treatment must either be extracted or maintained on a palliative care basis – maintaining oral hygiene as far as possible, while recognizing that gradual deterioration is likely, and that acute painful symptoms may occur with little warning. Such teeth, though unpredictable, may be maintained for many years. Their use as bridge abutments is best avoided if possible. It is questionable whether repeated scaling within a furcation is worthwhile if scaling failed at the first attempt.

Untreatable furcation-involved teeth, which are not in function or which repeatedly give rise to symptoms, should be extracted. Extraction should also be considered where an untreatable furcation lesion compromises the successful treatment of an adjacent tooth. For example, an upper premolar may be rendered untreatable by the close proximity of a mesial furcation lesion in the adjacent molar.

Prognosis

The preservation of connective tissue attachment around the roots of multirooted teeth depends on elimination of plaque, calculus and contaminated cementum and subsequent establishment of a gingival contour which can be maintained plaque-free. In the case of extensive lesions, this may be possible only if roots are resected to eliminate inaccessible areas of plaque accumulation and so prognosis may also depend on satisfactory endodontic treatment. However, limited resources preclude the wide application of such techniques and, therefore, many teeth are either extracted or maintained palliatively. In some cases, the risk of tooth loss may be *increased* by attempting root resection therapy. Finally, when several teeth are affected, one must be wary of planning treatment which is likely to be too extensive in relation to the expected benefits and which might preserve a dentition too complicated for satisfactory plaque control.

Prevention

As a fundamental principle, marginal disease should be diagnosed and treated early before attachment loss reaches furcation level. It is also important to recognize the potential for proximal furcation disease to arise adjacent to faulty restorations.

How to prevent restorations leading to furcation disease
1. Late diagnosis of proximal caries, with resulting large restorations, should be avoided.
2. Proximal contact areas should be maintained when restoring proximal surfaces.
3. Restoration margins should be supragingival, if possible.
4. Matrix bands should be adequately wedged and a check made for overhangs which should be removed during carving.
5. Restored surfaces should be checked for cervical fit using dental floss and a fine probe.

Periodontal–pulpal relationships

The purpose of this chapter is to outline the aetiology and management of lesions which may result from communication between the pulp space and the periodontium. Potential pathways for spread of infection are:

Pathways of infection
- Dentinal tubules.
- Lateral and accessory root canals.
- The apical foramen.
- Cracks and fracture lines.
- Iatrogenic perforations.

Classification and aetiology

The dental pulp has a limited capacity to respond to noxious stimuli. Loss of pulp vitality may be caused by the effects of caries, non-carious loss of tooth substance, restorative procedures and materials, thermal changes, trauma and the toxic effects of root surface plaque. In most cases, pulp changes reflect the cumulative effects of several stimuli.

Periodontal disease leading to secondary pulp involvement (Fig. 14.1). Gingival recession and root surface abrasion may expose dentinal tubules to the oral environment. Whether the resulting pulp changes are reversible or lead to progressive pulp necrosis will depend on the initial status of the pulp, and the severity and duration of noxious stimuli.

Within periodontal pockets, plaque bacteria and their toxins may come in contact with dentinal tubules where cementum has been affected by resorptive lesions or removed during treatment. Similarly, both periodontal lesions and therapy may involve lateral canals or fracture lines.

Pulp disease leading to secondary periodontal involvement (Fig. 14.2). Egress of bacteria, toxins and products of pulp necrosis from the apical foramen frequently results in an area of

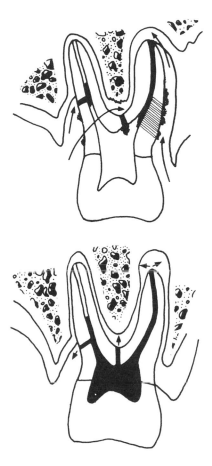

Fig. 14.1 Periodontal disease with secondary pulp involvement. Pulp may be affected via apical, lateral or accessory (furcation) canals or via dentine tubules.

Fig. 14.2 Pulp disease with secondary periodontal involvement via apical, lateral and accessory (furcation) canals.

destruction of periodontal ligament and adjacent bone. The same process may occur adjacent to lateral and accessory canals, fracture lines and iatrogenic perforations. The inflammatory process may lead to discharge of pus via a sinus tract through the periodontal ligament to the gingival margin inviting the misdiagnosis of a pocket of marginal periodontal origin. Another possible route for drainage is through the cortical plate apically, then subperiosteally to the gingival margin, without destruction of marginal periodontium. It may be possible by careful probing to distinguish these patterns of drainage.

'True' combined lesions (Fig. 14.3). In these cases there is no clear indication from history or examination of an aetiological link between the lesions of marginal periodontium and endodontic origin. A true combined lesion is, therefore, best

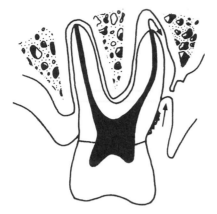

Fig. 14.3 True combined lesion. Lesions of apical and marginal origin communicate at the base of a deep periodontal pocket.

regarded as two separate lesions which have enlarged and merged.

Diagnosis

A careful history should be taken and followed by clinical examination, vitality tests and radiography. It is frequently impossible, however, to obtain a clear history for chronic, symptomless, periodontal–pulpal lesions. Diagnosis is generally easier during or just after an acute episode.

Clinical examination

One should be alerted to the possibility of periodontal–pulpal lesions by discoloured clinical crowns, sinuses, gross gingival exudate and probing depths which seem to be uncharacteristic of the general condition of the mouth.

When a lesion of endodontic origin spreads to involve a previously healthy marginal periodontium, probing may reveal a precipitous increase in probing depth atypical of the general level of periodontal destruction. Loss of pulp vitality should always be suspected when isolated, deep, narrow 'pockets' appear on facial tooth surfaces. Moreover, such root surfaces are likely to be relatively free of subgingival deposits unless the lesion is of long standing.

Pockets due to marginal periodontal disease usually possess a wide gingival orifice and deposits of calculus may be detected on the root surface. In addition, in established cases, probing depths tend to be greatest on proximal surfaces. Teeth are rarely affected in isolation.

Because of the cumulative effect of various noxious stimuli on the pulp, heavily restored teeth with significant attachment loss are more likely to be non-vital and exhibit combined lesions.

Vitality testing

The response of the pulp to vitality testing depends on an intact nerve supply, whereas vitality may be maintained by blood supply alone. Testing may be carried out electrically, thermally and by tactile stimulus with probe or bur. None of these tests is infallible and both false positive and false negative responses may be found. This is particularly likely in heavily restored teeth and in multirooted teeth.

Radiographic examination

This has been discussed in Chapter 6. A careful check should be made for widening of periodontal ligament space or loss of lamina dura, in addition to larger areas of periradicular rarefaction. Lesions may be masked by superimposition and their size tends to be underestimated. Lateral and accessory canals and fracture lines may be invisible. Furcation radiolucency may be endodontic in origin.

Correlation of diagnostic findings

A careful analysis of all available data will usually clarify the diagnosis. However, it may be impossible to establish the nature of a combined lesion particularly when of long duration. The patient should be advised and, where doubt exists, the lesion should be considered endodontic in origin.

Healing potential

The healing of endodontic lesions without marginal involvement is predictable if adequate endodontic treatment is carried out, and can be expected to result in regeneration of bone and periodontal ligament. This is because epithelium is normally excluded from the area. Regeneration of marginal periodontium, however, appears to be possible only to a very limited extent owing to the pathological and therapeutic alteration of tooth surface and the rapid migration of epithelium along the root surface from the gingival margin. The healing of combined lesions is, therefore, less predictable, as the proportion of periodontal destruction due to each process may be unclear and, in any case, chronic lesions of endodontic origin are likely to become plaque-infected and cementum pathologically altered. Whatever potential for regeneration may exist should be fully exploited, and so endodontic treatment should precede periodontal treatment. Periodontal treatment is destined to fail while infection of endodontic origin persists.

Treatment

Periodontal disease with secondary pulp involvement

Changes in the pulp secondary to periodontal disease may range from a mild reversible pulpitis to progressive necrosis.

Pulp hyperaemia may resolve as the periodontal disease is treated by removal of irritant deposits and by application of desensitizing agents to exposed dentine. If, however, periodontal disease leads to irreversible pulpitis or pulp necrosis, endodontic treatment should be carried out before periodontal treatment. Where attachment loss appears to involve the apex of a vital tooth, elective endodontic treatment should be considered prior to periodontal instrumentation. The prognosis for such teeth is usually poor.

Pulp disease with secondary periodontal involvement

Pulp disease will have progressed at least to partial necrosis and will necessitate endodontic treatment. Whether subsequent periodontal treatment is required will depend on the duration of communication with the gingival margin. When the duration of communication has been short (because of early diagnosis), plaque contamination of the root surface is less likely to have occurred and regeneration can be expected.

'True' combined lesions

Communication of long duration between lesions of endodontic and marginal origin is likely to result in accumulation of plaque and calculus with alteration of cementum over the entire root surface throughout the combined lesion. If the prognosis seems to justify treatment, such cases should first have endodontic treatment, to exploit fully any remaining regenerative potential. These lesions are likely also to require extensive débridement, possibly with surgical access.

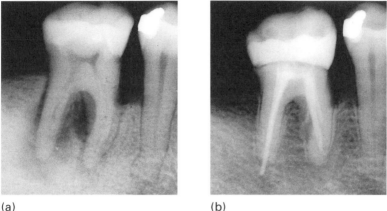

(a)   (b)

Fig. 14.4 (a) Molar with furcation and apical lesions arising from an infected pulp. (b) After endodontic treatment: the appearance of the root canal filling is less than ideal but the furcation lesion has healed. No periodontal treatment was required.

Furcation lesions

Accessory pulp canals are highly prevalent in the furcations of multirooted teeth. When a furcation lesion is diagnosed, vitality testing should be carried out and non-vital teeth treated endodontically, with a special search made of the floor of the pulp chamber for accessory canals. Furcation lesions of endodontic origin may be expected to heal if root canal therapy is carried out at an early stage (Fig. 14.4).

Iatrogenic lesions

These are usually endodontic in origin with secondary periodontal involvement, such as may occur with overfilling of root canals or perforation with root canal instruments or burs, often during post-crown preparation. It is important that any such problems are recognized early and the patient advised.

The prognosis for perforated roots is closely related to the size and position of the perforation. Small perforations in the apical third may be amenable to periradicular surgery. In the mid-third, perforations on the labial aspect will be accessible and should be repaired early. The prognosis is good if marginal communication is avoided. In the coronal third, marginal communication is likely to persist and a pocket may have to be accepted. Palatal and proximal surface perforations in the coronal two-thirds are likely to be inaccessible without removing excessive quantities of supporting bone.

Another form of post-crown failure is vertical root fracture. Leaching of root canal contents or bacterial contamination of the fracture line may lead to secondary periodontal involvement. The prognosis is usually hopeless.

Early onset periodontitis

Definitions

Early onset periodontitis (EOP) comprises a heterogeneous group of somewhat ill-defined forms of severe periodontitis affecting otherwise healthy children, adolescents and young adults. Its prevalence varies in geographically diverse populations. It is, for example, much commoner in African-Americans than in Caucasians. It is unclear whether the different forms of EOP represent variations in the phenotypic expression of a single disease, different stages of the same disease or separate disease entities. Indeed, there is no universally agreed terminology to describe the different manifestations of EOP described below.

Prepubertal periodontitis is said to occur in localized and generalized forms. Deciduous and permanent teeth may be involved. There is no agreement as to whether all periodontitis in the deciduous and mixed dentition should be given the 'prepubertal' label, or whether it should be reserved for disease beyond a certain level. Therefore, there are no agreed prevalence data for this condition.

Localized prepubertal periodontitis (LPP) is said to affect some but not all of the deciduous and/or permanent teeth and not to the extent of premature exfoliation. LPP is usually of little consequence to the affected child except that it may indicate a predisposition to EOP in the permanent dentition.

Generalized prepubertal periodontitis (GPP) is a very rare condition, affecting all the deciduous teeth and leading to premature exfoliation. It may be associated with a major systemic disorder such as neutropenia, hypophosphatasia, leucocyte adhesion deficiency, histiocytosis X, Chédiak-Higashi syndrome, Papillon-Lefèvre syndrome etc., and should, perhaps, be identified with the disorder rather than included as a form of EOP. Some cases, however, have been described in otherwise healthy children. The disease usually recurs in the permanent dentition.

Localized juvenile periodontitis (LJP) occurs in adolescents. It has its onset around puberty but may not be diagnosed until adulthood. Classically it affects only permanent incisors and first molars.

Generalized juvenile periodontitis (GJP) is a term used to describe cases of severe generalized periodontitis which are diagnosed in adolescence or in young adults with an arbitrary upper age limit of 35 years. In teenagers, GJP is much less common than LJP but its prevalence in young Caucasian adults under the age of 35 years appears to be about 1–2%, making it the commonest manifestation of EOP. Sometimes the expression 'generalized early onset periodontitis' is used instead of GJP, especially when referring to 20–35 year olds who no longer fit the 'juvenile' description.

Incidental attachment loss is a term used only in epidemiological studies to describe severe destructive lesions which affect isolated teeth without meeting the criteria for other forms of EOP. This category includes attachment loss adjacent to an impacted third molar.

Clinical features

Unlike chronic adult periodontitis, the prevalence and severity of which is broadly related to standards of oral hygiene, EOP may affect relatively clean as well as dirty mouths. When oral hygiene is poor, loss of periodontal support will be accompanied by frank gingivitis. On the other hand, in relatively clean mouths, gingivitis may be virtually absent, masking the presence of underlying destructive lesions. The condition is often brought to the patient's attention by the development of tooth mobility or migration, or the occurrence of a periodontal abscess, all signs of advanced destruction.

Aetiology

Different forms of EOP may coexist in the same family, and in some families the percentage of affected siblings approaches 50%. Although the primary hereditary defect is unknown, this seems to be manifest as a gross imbalance of host–parasite equilibrium so that, following a short period of exposure to small amounts of plaque, perhaps containing specific pathogens, destructive lesions develop.

A variety of host response defects, including inherited defects in circulating polymorphonuclear neutrophil granulocytes (PMNs) has been described. It must be stressed, however, that there appears to be no single characteristic defect responsible for EOP, and many affected individuals fail to demonstrate any abnormality.

Subgingival plaque is often present only as a thin Gram-negative layer, loosely attached to the tooth surface, in contrast to adult chronic periodontitis where a comparatively thick subgingival flora is present. Subgingival calculus is often absent in EOP.

Treatment of EOP

All forms of periodontitis, including EOP, share a common approach to treatment: the establishment of good oral hygiene and thorough subgingival débridement, with surgical access if necessary. Better, more predictable results are obtained from treatment of LJP than GJP. Adjunctive, antimicrobial therapy may be employed (see Chapter 16) but is more likely to be effective in cases of LJP than GJP.

Features specific to localized juvenile periodontitis

Among all forms of periodontitis, LJP is probably the best characterized and displays the least heterogeneity. Initially, first permanent molars and/or permanent incisors are affected but one or more of the adjacent premolar and molar surfaces may also be involved (Fig. 15.1) and, ultimately, progression to GJP may occur. The incisor/molar pattern of involvement may be a reflection of their earlier eruption times and the fact that they have been exposed longer to the oral environment.

In Caucasians, the prevalence of LJP is roughly 0.1% compared to a prevalence rate of about 1.0–3.0% in ethnic negroid populations. An American study of 11 007 14–17 year olds suggests that LJP may affect white females more frequently than white males and black males more commonly than black females, in both cases by a factor of 3:1.

The subgingival flora of LJP has a variable composition and may include any of the putative pathogens described in Table 3.1. However, *Actinobacillus actinomycetemcomitans (A. a.)*, a capnophilic, non-motile rod, is isolated more frequently and often in greater proportions than from adult periodontitis lesions. This organism possesses numerous virulence factors. A potent leucotoxin, for example, is produced by many strains of *A. a.* causing lysis of PMNs and monocytes. Furthermore, there

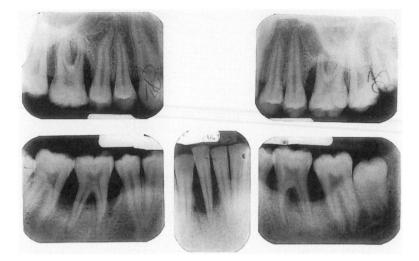

Fig. 15.1 Juvenile periodontitis affecting the lower right central incisor and the first molars and lower second molars in an 18 year old.

is some evidence, not fully substantiated, that *A. a.* may be capable of invading pocket soft tissues. There is usually a lower proportional recovery of *A. a.* from older GJP subjects, whose flora comprises a wider range of pathogens.

In spite of the obvious rapidity with which attachment loss has taken place, the response of the tissues to treatment is generally good. Rapid healing can often be observed, and more bone regeneration may occur within angular bone defects than might be expected following treatment of adult periodontitis. These observations might suggest that LJP is often 'burned out' by the time of diagnosis and treatment.

A number of studies have been carried out showing that systemic antimicrobial therapy immediately after thorough mechanical débridement may give better results than instrumentation alone, whether non-surgical or surgical. This suggests that *A. a.* may be difficult to eradicate by instrumentation alone from periodontal tissues which it is thought to invade. Many drug regimens have been tested, including tetracycline for 14 days or a combination of amoxicillin with metronidazole for 7 days (see Chapter 16).

Although the benefits of systemic antimicrobial drug therapy are well documented, several investigators have reported excellent results from conventional treatment without antibiotics in patients followed up for several years.

16

Chemical antimicrobial pocket therapy

Antimicrobial chemotherapy may be used to support traditional pocket therapy, and may be employed topically within the periodontal pocket or systemically.

Before considering their use, it is essential to recognize that dental bacterial plaque is extremely resistant to chemical antimicrobial agents because of the 'biofilm effect'.

> Plaque exists as a 'biofilm' composed of extracellular bacterial polymers with salivary and gingival exudate products forming a matrix within which bacteria are embedded. The biofilm protects bacteria from antimicrobial agents and must be disrupted physically before these drugs can be effective.

Hence, antimicrobial agents should be employed *immediately after* thorough mechanical débridement.

Systemic antimicrobial agents in the treatment of periodontitis

Clear indications exist for the use of systemic antimicrobial drugs in the treatment of periodontal abscesses and acute necrotizing ulcerative gingivitis. The purpose of this section, however, is to discuss their role in the management of chronic periodontitis for which, in recent years, many drug regimens have been suggested. In fact, there are very few well designed prospective randomized placebo-controlled trials incorporating long-term follow up on which to base rational treatment decisions. Nevertheless, a consensus has been reached on the following points.

> Systemic antimicrobial drug therapy should be reserved for the small minority of patients who, in spite of maintaining good plaque control, have proved unresponsive to conventional mechanical therapy, i.e. those with very aggressive forms of periodontitis. Antimicrobial drugs should be

prescribed in conjunction with further instrumentation to support the host defence system by suppressing subgingival pathogens that evade the mechanical débridement process.

A brief profile of the most commonly used drugs is given below.

Tetracyclines are broad-spectrum bacteriostatic antibiotics. Tetracycline hydrochloride, and its more expensive but more readily absorbed semisynthetic derivatives, doxycycline and minocycline, accumulate within the pocket and achieve gingival fluid concentrations which are two to five times higher than serum levels. Tetracyclines, furthermore, inhibit host-derived collagenases and other matrix metalloproteinases by a mechanism independent of their antimicrobial activity, and may, therefore, suppress connective tissue breakdown. Common adverse effects include gastrointestinal intolerance, *Candida* superinfection and interaction with oral contraceptives. Tetracycline should not be given in pregnancy or childhood because of its potential to stain mineralizing tooth substance.

Metronidazole is a bactericidal compound which is effective against strict anaerobes but not, *in vitro*, against facultative anaerobes or capnophilic organisms such as *Actinobacillus actinomycetemcomitans (A. a.)*. Adverse effects include gastrointestinal intolerance, metallic taste and, when alcohol is taken within 24 hours of drug ingestion, a range of unpleasant symptoms due to accumulation of acetaldehyde in the blood. Metronidazole should not be taken in pregnancy or by nursing mothers. Various drug interactions may also occur.

Amoxicillin is a semisynthetic penicillin possessing bactericidal activity against a broad spectrum of bacteria. To be effective in the treatment of chronic periodontitis it must be combined with clavulanic acid or metronidazole. Clavulanic acid (a β-lactamase blocker), extends its range of activity to include β-lactamase-producing bacteria. Synergistic action against *A. actinomycetemcomitans* is observed when amoxicillin is combined with metronidazole. Amoxicillin may give rise to hypersensitivity reactions ranging from a minor skin rash to anaphylactic shock.

Numerous drugs, including those listed above, have been used singly, in combination or serially in the treatment of various manifestations of periodontitis, with mixed results. There is limited information on the optimum dosage or dosing interval and the duration of therapy has varied from a few days to several weeks.

Since periodontitis is a mixed infection in which the predominant pathogens are difficult to identify, and since individual isolates may have different drug sensitivities, it seems unlikely that expensive laboratory tests would help the clinician to make a more informed choice of antibiotic for individual cases. In due course, once a large enough data set is obtained from clinical trials of systemic antimicrobial agents, and a hierarchy of drugs and protocols is available, it should be possible to take advantage of microbiological tests.

In the meantime, based on the research data currently available, the drug regimen of choice, as an adjunct to thorough subgingival instrumentation, would appear to be:

Metronidazole 200 mg three times daily for 7 days
with
Amoxicillin 500 mg three times daily for 7 days

As well as achieving relatively good clinical results, compared to other drug therapies, this drug combination is highly successful at eliminating the major periodontal pathogens, *A. actinomycetemcomitans* and *Porphyromonas gingivalis*. Some research workers take the view that these organisms are exogenous pathogens, and that disease will recur unless they are eliminated.

For patients allergic to penicillin the suggested regimen is:

Tetracycline 250 mg four times daily for 14 days
or
Metronidazole 200 mg three times daily for 10 days

Readers are urged to recognize that, due to the widespread use of antibiotics, a large and increasing number of important human pathogens are resistant to them. This has become a serious medical, economic and public health problem. Antibiotic therapy for chronic periodontitis should, therefore, be used with great restraint and only after conventional measures, including specialist referral, have been undertaken. Above all, antibiotic therapy should never be a substitute for plaque control instruction and thorough subgingival instrumentation.

Pocket irrigation

Chlorhexidine, although safe and effective as an inhibitor of supragingival plaque, does not, when used *as a mouthwash*, enter periodontal pockets and is, therefore, ineffective in the treatment of periodontitis. Numerous studies, however, have been carried out to test the efficacy of *pocket irrigation* with chlorhexidine as an adjunct to root instrumentation in the treatment of periodontitis. These studies have evaluated different methods of irrigation: by syringe; by pulsated jet delivery; and as coolants during ultrasonic subgingival scaling. Generally, results have been disappointing. Where an improvement in gingival conditions has been demonstrated, this has been confined to the marginal tissues and may be attributable to the effect of the chlorhexidine effluent on *supragingival* plaque at the point of delivery.

Several other antimicrobial agents have been tested as pocket irrigants, but none has shown promise.

Chlorhexidine's failure to have a significant effect on the subgingival microflora may be partly attributed to its inability to influence preformed plaque and partly to the lack of time for adsorption of the chlorhexidine to the subgingival root surface and soft-tissue pocket wall. Thus an effective concentration of the agent within the pocket would not be established and maintained. The need to maintain optimal concentrations of antimicrobial agents for use in periodontal pockets has led to the testing of various sustained- and controlled-release delivery systems.

Sustained and controlled local drug delivery

Sustained-release subgingival drug delivery is currently achieved by syringe application of biodegradable metronidazole gel or tetracycline ointment after which the drug level decreases exponentially at a rate directly proportional to its pocket concentration. Controlled-release delivery achieves high drug concentrations in the pocket for a prolonged period of time. This involves the insertion of non-resorbable tetracycline-containing ethylene vinyl acetate fibre, or a resorbable hydrolysed gelatin matrix which contains chlorhexidine. These are attractive concepts which, compared to systemic drug delivery, offer the following advantages.

Advantages of sustained or controlled local drug delivery
- Higher drug concentrations are achievable.
- Drugs unsuitable for systemic administration may be used.
- Dosing is not dependent on patient compliance.
- Bacterial resistance at remote body sites may be avoided.
- Superinfection at remote body sites may be avoided.
- Gastrointestinal intolerance is avoided.

Metronidazole gel and minocycline ointment are marketed in disposable syringe applicators as adjuncts to mechanical débridement of deep pockets. Preliminary research findings reveal that effective antimicrobial concentrations are maintained for up to one day but only modest clinical benefits have been observed. Long-term efficacy and possible adverse effects, such as selection of resistant organisms, have yet to be determined.

Tetracycline-containing monolithic fibres of ethylene vinyl acetate will maintain a high concentration of tetracycline in the periodontal pocket for several days. By this method, drug levels in the pocket may be achieved which are up to 100 times greater than those obtained by systemic administration of a 250 mg dose of tetracycline. Unfortunately, this mode of treatment is time-consuming. It can be uncomfortable for the patient and involves the use of cyanoacrylate to seal the fibre in the pocket.

Chlorhexidine-containing 'chips', suitable for insertion into pockets, are currently under investigation. Bacteriological studies, conducted after long-term use of chlorhexidine mouthwash, have shown that bacterial mutation and selection of resistant strains does not occur. This could give chlorhexidine an advantage over topical antibiotic agents where the development of bacterial resistance is potentially a problem.

Sustained and controlled local drug delivery systems have a potential role in the treatment of patients with excellent plaque control, where one or two sites have failed to respond to thorough débridement. However, so far there is limited evidence of their efficacy and cost effectiveness when used for that purpose.

Gingival deficiency

Attached gingiva is well suited to withstand frictional stresses from the passage of food and the use of the toothbrush, and to dissipate pull from the lip and cheek musculature. Its width (height) in the developing dentition is determined by hereditary factors, including growth of the alveolar process, position of teeth within the arch and location of fraenal insertion. Thus, there is great variation in width of attached gingiva between and within individuals. Occasionally there is no attached gingiva at all, usually because of high fraenal insertion (Fig. 17.1). Attached gingival width, therefore, may be inherently deficient, but it can also be reduced by gingival recession (Fig. 17.2) or increased as occlusal attrition and compensatory overeruption occur.

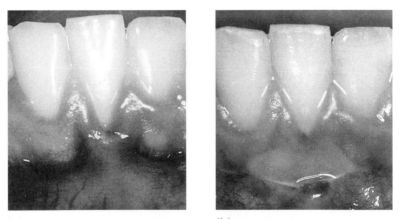

(a)   (b)

Fig. 17.1 Gingival augmentation. Left, a high fraenal attachment reduces access for toothbrushing; right, after free gingival graft surgery. Note, however, that toothbrushing habits have not altered and gingivitis is still present.

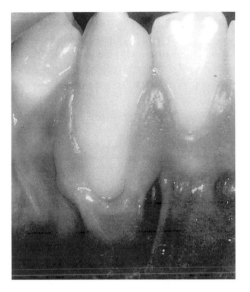

Fig. 17.2 Clinically healthy gingiva in spite of unfavourable mucogingival relationships at the 43. The patient has learned to overcome the difficulty of cleaning the cervical portion of this tooth.

Aetiology of recession

Aetiology of recession

Tooth position	Occlusal trauma
Inflammation	Removable prostheses
Toothbrush trauma	Orthodontic tooth movement
Pernicious oral habits	Subgingival restoration
	margins

Tooth position. Teeth which are prominent buccally or lingually are predisposed to gingival recession. The alveolar crest may be located at a more apical level forming a bony dehiscence, and the remainder of the root may be covered by a *thin* layer of attached gingival tissue with a reduced capacity to withstand inflammatory or traumatic insults.

Inflammation. Gingival recession commonly accompanies plaque-induced chronic periodontal disease. It may occur on any tooth surface and is probably the commonest explanation for *interdental* gingival recession.

Toothbrush trauma. The toothbrush is a frequent cause of recession affecting buccal and lingual surfaces. Presumably, the force applied, the speed and frequency of brushing, the texture of the brush and abrasion from toothpaste are important factors. Toothbrush trauma is usually associated with good buccal and lingual plaque control, gingival health and smooth, highly-polished tooth surfaces. Cervical abrasion cavities may be present.

Pernicious oral habits. Children or adolescents may exhibit gingival ulceration and recession due to repeated injury from the habitual use of fingernails, pencils, etc.

Occlusal trauma. Tooth movement may occur as an adaptive response to occlusal trauma. Depending on the nature of the forces, this may result in migration or mobility and, perhaps, in bony dehiscence, which is often followed by gingival recession. Trauma from occlusion may also take the form of gingival surface injury. Thus, excessive incisor overlap may allow upper incisors to injure the lower labial gingivae or lower incisors to injure the upper palatal gingivae. Food will impinge against the gingival margin during mastication, and bruxist habits may perpetuate the soft-tissue trauma.

Removable prostheses. Unless adequately tooth supported, removable prostheses may impinge upon gingival tissue and precipitate recession. Alternatively, prostheses may cause tooth movement and subsequent recession. Some of the tissue damage may also be attributable to the inflammatory changes produced by increased plaque accumulation beneath the denture.

Orthodontic tooth movement. When a tooth is moved accidentally or unavoidably through the buccal or lingual cortical plate, causing a bony dehiscence, gingival recession may ensue.

Subgingival restoration margins. Because of the potential for plaque accumulation, restoration margins, placed subgingivally, may cause inflammatory alterations in the adjacent gingiva leading to recession, especially if the gingival tissue is thin.

Pathogenesis of recession

Where gingival tissue is thin, an inflammatory or traumatic lesion may occupy and degrade the entire thickness of connective tissue. Epithelial cells will tend to proliferate into the degraded connective tissue, forming interconnecting cords of epithelium between the oral and pocket epithelia, and making connective tissue recovery impossible. This is followed by subsidence of the epithelial surface and 'shrinkage' of marginal gingiva. It follows that thick marginal gingiva will be less susceptible to recession.

Even when the entire width of attached gingiva has been destroyed, marginal tissue will usually continue to keratinize at the orifice of the gingival sulcus, creating a narrow zone of free gingiva. This occurs, not in response to functional demands, but due to morphogenetic stimuli from the underlying periodontal ligament.

Clinical significance of a minimal width of attached gingiva

It has been shown from numerous experimental studies that:

1. With good plaque control, marginal inflammation will not occur, irrespective of the presence or absence of attached gingiva.
2. If plaque does accumulate, the inflammatory lesion in the marginal soft tissue is not enhanced in cases where the zone of attached gingiva is very narrow or missing altogether.
3. Gingival recession is *not* more likely to occur in areas with very little gingiva than in areas of considerable width.

Thus, there is no minimum required width of attached gingiva. Furthermore, the presence of a deficient band of attached gingiva should not give cause for concern *unless* the abnormal tissue morphology prohibits satisfactory plaque control, leading to chronic periodontal disease. Particular difficulty with oral hygiene may be experienced when a fraenum is attached at the soft tissue margin (see Fig. 17.1). The patient may modify his toothbrushing technique to avoid traumatizing the non-keratinized alveolar mucosa and fail to achieve complete plaque removal, leading to inflammatory changes with further recession and/or pocket formation: gingival recession is likely to cease when thicker mucosa is reached, but if plaque accumulation persists, periodontal breakdown may continue with the development of pockets.

Management of gingival deficiency

In the developing dentition of preteenage children, lower incisors are often displaced buccally with an associated reduction in width of free and attached gingiva. However, as the child matures, spontaneous tooth realignment may occur and be accompanied by coronal regrowth of free gingiva. Thus, although there is no increase in width of attached gingiva, there is a dimensional improvement in keratinized gingiva which should facilitate plaque control.

Where gingivitis or periodontitis occurs in areas of minimal gingival width, the first line of treatment involves instruction in an efficient but atraumatic brushing technique and, if necessary, scaling and root planing. The single-tufted toothbrush is often helpful. In the majority of cases, no further treatment is necessary (see Fig. 17.2).

Where gingival recession is present, all aetiological factors should be eliminated as far as possible. This means that, in addition to teaching an effective, atraumatic cleaning technique, other sources of trauma should be eliminated; and displaced, migrated or hypermobile teeth may require stabilization within the arch.

When, in spite of careful instruction, patients remain unable to perform adequate oral hygiene owing to adverse soft tissue morphology, mucogingival surgery should be considered. There are essentially two options.

1. Gingival augmentation surgery to create a deepened vestibule and sufficient width of attached gingiva, apical to the original mucogingival junction, to allow toothbrushing without discomfort. This approach is applicable mainly to teeth with an inherent lack of attached gingiva and minimal or no root exposure rather than to those affected by significant gingival recession. Gingival augmentation is usually achieved by the free gingival graft technique (Figs 17.1 and 17.3).

2. Root coverage surgery for teeth affected by gingival recession. Plaque control is facilitated by restoring a layer of keratinized gingiva to the root surface and by re-creating the gingival margin at the same level as adjacent teeth. Root coverage surgery may also be employed primarily to address aesthetic concerns or to treat root hypersensitivity.

Gingival augmentation

Biological rationale of the free gingival graft. The potential for epithelium to keratinize depends, not on functional demands, but mainly on morphogenetic stimuli from the connective tissue to which the epithelium is attached. Hence, a transplant of keratinized mucosa, when located within the alveolar mucosa (an environment where keratinization is normally absent), will retain its surface characteristics owing to the stimulus of the underlying transplanted connective tissue. This is the rationale behind the free gingival graft procedure.

Free gingival graft – outline of the technique (see Fig. 17.3). An incision is made at the mucogingival line and a mucosal flap is reflected leaving a thin layer of periosteum on the alveolar

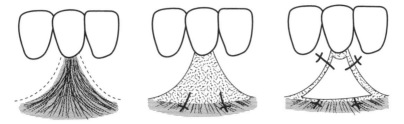

Fig. 17.3 Free gingival graft for gingival augmentation: left, the incision (broken line); centre, suturing the flap; and right, suturing the graft.

process. The flap margin should be sutured to its base. A foil template of the recipient site is produced and transferred to the premolar region of the palate, just behind the rugae, about 3 mm from the gingival margins of these teeth. An incision is made round the foil to a depth of 2 mm, i.e. extending to the full thickness of the mucosa but without including a significant amount of submucosa. The foil is removed and the graft tissue dissected out. Any adherent fatty or glandular tissue should be scraped from the graft before suturing to the recipient site. Pressure is then applied to expel blood from between the graft and its recipient bed prior to application of a periodontal dressing. The donor site is protected by an acrylic plate, manufactured from a preoperative impression. Dressing and sutures are removed after one week and the patient advised to avoid brushing the area of the graft for 2–4 weeks. Chlorhexidine mouthwash is used during this time.

Free gingival graft – wound healing. Survival of the graft in the first two postoperative days is solely dependent on a plasmatic circulation, i.e. diffusion of nutrients from the host bed. Thereafter, a capillary network extends into the graft. Although graft epithelium usually desquamates, it is recolonized by epithelium from adjacent tissues, with keratinization occurring in 4 weeks.

Root coverage surgery

A variety of techniques is available. All involve grafting; either free grafts which, until they integrate with host tissue, have no blood supply, or pedicle grafts which retain their own blood supply. For pedicle grafts to be considered, there must be an adequate zone of adjacent gingiva, either mesial, distal or apical to the defect. Ideally, this donor tissue should be thick enough to be itself resistant to recession. Otherwise, a layer of transplanted palatal connective tissue should be placed under the pedicle(s). Before root coverage is attempted, the exposed root should be thoroughly débrided and, if prominent, can be ground slightly flatter to reduce its exposure to traumatic forces and to minimize the mesiodistal width of the avascular recipient bed.

Free (epithelialized) gingival graft. This technique is similar to the one just described for gingival augmentation. However, instead of placing the graft on a bed composed entirely of periosteum, apical to the alveolar crest, it is placed directly over the exposed root, overlapping the adjacent surgically exposed periosteum both laterally and apically by at least 3 mm, thereby tapping a source of nourishment to sustain the portion of graft which lies on the denuded root surface.

Free subepithelial connective tissue graft. After first excising the sulcular epithelium from the marginal gingiva of the affected root, the marginal soft tissue is undermined by sharp dissection, creating a pouch or 'envelope' at least 3 mm deep. A connective tissue graft is harvested from the palate by a 'trapdoor' approach and placed half in and half out of the envelope. The protruding portion covers the exposed root while the 'sheathed' part is nourished by the periosteum below and the undersurface of the gingiva above. Survival of the graft tissue, projecting from the envelope and lying on the denuded root surface, is dependent on collateral circulation. Free connective tissue grafts can also be placed beneath the pedicle grafts described below to obtain enhanced gingival thickness over the recipient root.

Laterally positioned flap. This is a pedicle graft obtained from an adjacent tooth. Recession at the donor site may complicate this procedure (Fig. 17.4(a)).

Double pedicle flap. Interradicular soft tissue is obtained from either side of the affected tooth and the pair of obliquely repositioned pedicles sutured together over the root (Fig. 17.4(b)).

Coronally positioned flap. Gingiva still present apical to the recession defect is advanced coronally to cover the root. With a shallow recession defect this can be achieved by creating a flap from a semilunar incision parallel to the curvature of the gingival margin and about 3 mm apical to it (Fig. 17.4(c)). Alternatively, two apically divergent vertical releasing incisions are made (Fig. 17.4(d)).

Coronally positioned flap with GTR. Recently the principles of guided tissue regeneration (GTR) for maximizing the formation of new connective tissue attachment (see Chapter 12) have been successfully applied to root coverage with a coronally

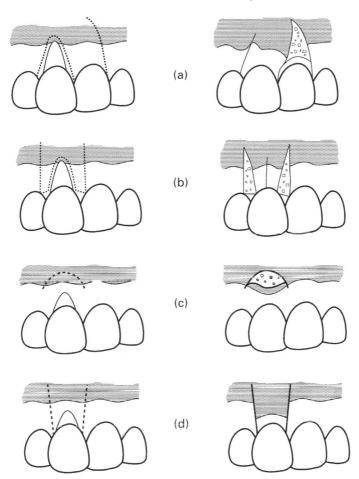

Fig. 17.4 Root coverage with pedicle grafts: (a) laterally positioned flap; (b) double pedicle flap; (c) coronally positioned flap from a semilunar incision; (d) coronally positioned flap from 2 vertical incisions.

positioned flap. A barrier membrane with malleable titanium 'ribs', to create a space underneath for tissue formation, is sutured in place over the exposed root and the flap is advanced coronally to cover it. There are, however, significant drawbacks. These include the cost of the materials, the need for a second operation to remove the membrane and reduced predictability of complete root coverage.

Root coverage – wound healing. Clinical studies have shown that these procedures achieve, on average, about 75% root coverage and, in approximately 50% of cases, complete coverage is obtained. Procedures which incorporate connective tissue grafts appear to give the best results. Narrow recession defects are easiest to treat. It is likely that some new connective tissue attachment will form in the apical and lateral parts of the recession defect while an epithelial attachment will form in the coronal and mid-buccal portion of the root.

In spite of its predictability, mucogingival surgery has a limited role in the acquisition and maintenance of periodontal health. It should be reserved for cases where, because of an unfavourable soft tissue morphology, good plaque control cannot be achieved and gingival health secured, and for patients with aesthetic problems due to gingival recession.

Occlusal therapy

Introduction

Occlusal therapy in periodontics may be defined as any procedure which, by altering the direction, magnitude or distribution of occlusal forces, will reduce trauma or stabilize a tooth which is mobile or subject to migration. This is achieved usually by reshaping occlusal surfaces (occlusal adjustment) or by increasing the tooth's resistance to applied force (splinting), or occasionally by orthodontics. The intention of this chapter is to put occlusal therapy in proper perspective in relation to periodontal disease and, therefore, only a brief description will be given of a few selected techniques of occlusal treatment.

Occlusal therapy may be irreversible: most forms of occlusal adjustment and some forms of splinting involve destruction of tooth substance. So far as periodontal problems are concerned, it should be reserved for a few well-defined situations.

Indications

The main indications for occlusal therapy are as follows:

1. Progressive occlusal trauma.
   a) surface injury (e.g. deep traumatic overbite).
   b) injury to the supporting structures.
2. Tooth hypermobility (if it interferes with patient comfort or prevents adequate root instrumentation).
3. Tooth migration.

Of course, occlusal therapy may be necessary prior to restorative treatment, but is intended primarily to facilitate the construction of satisfactory restorations and control the risk of technical failure, rather than to benefit the periodontium directly.

In every case an occlusal aetiology must be demonstrable for occlusal therapy to be effective. Failure to observe this rule may result in unjustified mutilation of the occlusion. Tooth mobility, for example, is an inevitable consequence of marginal periodontitis, sooner or later, and it may persist even after successful treatment to arrest periodontal disease. A belief that any tooth mobility is unacceptable or necessarily a sign of poor prognosis may lead, either to overtreatment by means of occlusal therapy, or even to unnecessary tooth extraction. Most tooth mobility should be regarded as a sign of a reduced periodontium and appropriate steps should be taken to ensure control of inflammatory periodontal disease as a first priority. Only if mobility interferes with patient comfort or appears to be increasing in the absence of ongoing inflammatory periodontal disease, should occlusal therapy be considered, subject to the demonstration of a relevant occlusal abnormality.

Occlusal adjustment

Occlusal adjustment involves an alteration to the occluding surfaces of teeth to achieve stable, non-traumatic, contact relationships in maximum intercuspation and in all functional excursive contact positions. Forces transmitted through the teeth should, as far as possible, be directed parallel to their long axes. This is particularly important in cases of reduced periodontal support.

Occlusal adjustment is usually achieved by grinding or sometimes by restorations. In periodontics, the aim is to eliminate certain occlusal contacts: those which interfere with the free gliding movement of the mandible causing inappropriate stress distribution; or those which subject the periodontal tissues of an individual tooth or group of teeth to excessive load relative to remaining periodontal support. As a first step in this process, a careful analysis of the occlusion must be made. It is good practice never to start an occlusal adjustment where doubt exists that the desired result can be achieved. Trial adjustments on mounted study casts can be carried out to assess the feasibility of occlusal adjustment.

It is not sufficient simply to eliminate interfering contacts unless a stable occlusion is produced; one in which drifting or tipping cannot occur or new interferences develop. If adjustment causes instability, splinting may be necessary. If, for example, the incisal edge of a lower anterior tooth is ground to eliminate a protrusive interference and to transfer the load to other teeth, there will be loss of centric contact and overeruption of that tooth or its opponent. Eventually it will re-establish its previous unsatisfactory occlusal relationship with its opponent in the upper arch. Protrusive interferences, therefore, can be eliminated and stable occlusal relationships produced only by grinding the palatal slopes and incisal edges of upper incisors and canines, and this may be aesthetically unacceptable. This is particularly true in cases of increased overbite. Splinting, therefore, is often a more appropriate means of occlusal therapy for anterior teeth.

Splinting

Splinting is the procedure by which a tooth's resistance to an applied force is increased by joining it to a neighbouring tooth or teeth. Splints may be classified as temporary or permanent, fixed or removable, rigid or flexible, intracoronal or extracoronal.

Splints are used in periodontics principally to stabilize anterior teeth which are subject to migration, or to retain anterior teeth which have been realigned. They may also be used to stabilize teeth which are so mobile that they interfere with patient comfort especially during mastication. There is a wide variety of splints in current use. None has met with universal acceptance and, in most cases, documented evidence of clinical longevity is lacking. Some of the more popular types are described below.

Composite resin-retained splints

Unless used in great bulk, composite resin lacks sufficient trans verse strength to splint mobile teeth. However, it may be used as a cementing medium for 'Rochette'- or 'Maryland'-type splints. These comprise custom-made cast bars in non-precious alloy, fitting against the lingual surfaces of teeth. The composite cement engages etched tooth enamel on one side and, on the other, either countersunk perforations in the bar (Rochette technique) or a sand-blasted metal fitting surface.

The Rochette and Maryland techniques are applicable mainly to lower anterior teeth. They are suitable for upper anterior teeth only where occlusal relationships will accommodate the necessary thickness of metal. Otherwise preparation of palatal or opposing tooth surfaces will be necessary. Evidence which is mainly anecdotal suggests that failure of retention is not uncommon. Whereas a Rochette splint can easily be removed if cementation failure occurs, it is usually impossible to remove a Maryland-type splint intact. Thus, an important consideration in the choice of resin-retained splint should be its ease of repair.

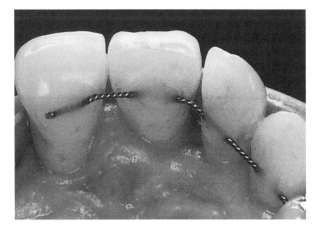

Fig. 18.1 Multistrand wire splint.

Braided multistrand wire, in use for almost 25 years for fixed orthodontic retention, can also be employed to splint mobile teeth. It is adapted to the lingual tooth surfaces on a plaster model, transferred to the mouth, and cemented to the cingulum region of each tooth (Fig. 18.1). Each tooth retains slight independent mobility, which may be advantageous in the maintenance of a structurally normal periodontium. These splints are inexpensive to fabricate and easy to repair. The composite resin does not cover a large expanse of lingual tooth surface and can be utilized in the upper anterior region even in cases of slightly increased overbite (Fig. 18.2). These features make multistrand wire the material of choice both for splinting mobile teeth and preventing tooth migration.

The stresses to which the composite resin cementing medium is subjected in all types of resin-retained splint are considerable, especially when the splinted teeth have little independent support and are inherently hypermobile. Where possible, therefore, occlusal interferences should be eliminated in order to distribute load more evenly.

Linked full veneer crowns

Linked full veneer crowns are indicated mainly for splinting upper anterior teeth in patients with an overbite so deep that a resin-retained splint cannot be constructed (Fig. 18.2(c) and (d)). This is also the technique of choice for splinting heavily restored or otherwise unsightly teeth. Serious consideration, however,

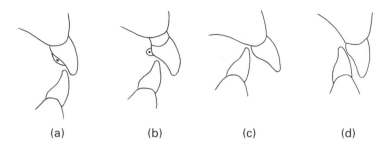

(a)   (b)   (c)   (d)

Fig. 18.2 (a) Normal overbite and (b) slightly increased overbite with gingival recession, both suitable for resin-bonded extracoronal wire retainers. (c) and (d) Deep overbites preclude extracoronal wire retention.

should be given to avoiding a full-coverage splint when teeth are intact, since large amounts of tooth substance must be destroyed to accommodate metal and porcelain and there is a significant risk of pulp damage due to the technical difficulty of making multiple parallel preparations. A further drawback is the added potential for plaque accumulation at the crown margin adjacent to the gingiva in patients susceptible to periodontitis.

Removable acrylic occlusal splints (bite planes)

In cases where a deep overbite, involving sound teeth, precludes either of the foregoing methods, the construction of an acrylic occlusal splint as a night-guard may be considered. This consists of a simple acrylic splint with incisor edge cover, retained by Adams cribs on molar teeth. It is worn at night to stabilize teeth which, during the day, possess a potential to drift forwards. This type of splint is also useful where large spaces are present between upper incisors, preventing the construction of an aesthetically acceptable fixed splint.

Since day-time wear is impractical, these splints are unsuitable for stabilizing teeth which possess an unacceptable level of mobility.

Removable partial dentures

In the management of tooth mobility and migration, the advantage of a removable partial denture is often limited to its effect in redistributing masticatory load rather than to any splinting effect of the rigid denture base components. Consideration of a partial denture for this purpose needs to be weighed against its potential to enhance plaque accumulation and thus compromise the periodontium further.

Anterior tooth migration

Anterior tooth migration is a common complaint of patients presenting with periodontal disease. Its management embraces many aspects of occlusal therapy and will now be considered in more detail.

Migration may be a sequel to tooth loss or the adoption of a parafunctional habit. In some patients, the resistance offered even by a normal healthy periodontium is barely sufficient to prevent the forces acting on the teeth from causing migration. In these cases, drifting may occur as soon as inflammatory destruction of supporting tissues (periodontitis) begins. In other cases, tooth migration may be a late feature of periodontitis. Patients' thresholds of perception of changes in anterior tooth position and their degree of anxiety about them vary widely, and migration may be noted before a significant increase in tooth mobility or other signs of periodontal disease.

Aetiology

The following is a list of common aetiological factors:

1. Marginal periodontitis.
2. Periapical osteitis.
3. Loss of adjacent teeth.
4. Loss of posterior teeth with distal drift of part of the anterior segment.
5. Centric interferences: either a premature contact between the affected anterior tooth and its opponent or, more commonly, a posterior deflective contact creating an anterior path of closure.
6. Protrusive interferences.
7. Parafunctional habits such as bruxism, lip biting, nail biting, pipe smoking and playing a wind instrument.

Treatment

The first priority in treatment is the removal of aetiological factors before corrective treatment is attempted. The list of possible management options will, therefore, include:

1. Periodontal and endodontic treatment.
2. Elimination of parafunctional habits.
3. Monitoring tooth positions with study casts.
4. Occlusal adjustment.
5. Replacement of missing teeth.
6. Splinting without realignment.
7. Orthodontic realignment and splinting.
8. Repositioning by crown construction.
9. Composite augmentation to reduce spaces.
10. Extraction and prosthesis.

The initial aim of periodontal therapy will be the establishment of periodontal health with the arrest of attachment loss. Where infrabony pockets are present, bone-fill may be achieved and marginal support, thereby, improved. Endodontic treatment, where required, should improve periapical support.

These measures alone may be sufficient to achieve tooth stability and reduce the risk of further migration. Therefore, if the new tooth position is acceptable to the patient, reference casts may be obtained to monitor tooth position. Where doubt persists concerning tooth stability, splinting may be employed as described earlier in this chapter, although it may be advisable to realign the tooth first.

Where the position of the migrated tooth is aesthetically unacceptable, orthodontic treatment should be considered, and will be simple to accomplish so long as space is available for realignment. Frequently, however, upper anterior tooth migration is accompanied by anterior migration of lower teeth and/or by extrusion of the migrated teeth or their opponents. Orthodontic therapy will then involve appliance therapy in both arches and/or intrusion of overerupted teeth. Very occasionally, it may be possible to create space for retraction of upper anterior teeth by occlusal adjustment to stabilize the mandible in a more distal occlusal position. This, of course, will be possible only where there is a posterior deflective contact.

After realignment, permanent splinting is almost always necessary and an acceptable means by which this may be achieved should be determined before orthodontic therapy commences.

Tooth realignment, by means of artificial crowns on realigned posts and cores following endodontic treatment, is usually only possible where lower anterior teeth have not invaded the desired anterior tooth position. It is essential to check that a stable position can be found for the new crowns, preferably by the use of mounted diagnostic casts. If a stable position cannot be found, some means of permanent retention will be necessary.

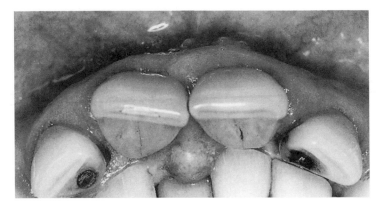

Fig. 18.3 Deep traumatic overbite.

Deep traumatic overbite

Clinical features (Fig. 18.3)

In an 'ideal' relationship, the incisal edges of the lower incisors and the cinguli of the upper incisors provide the centric stops necessary to maintain tooth position and prevent overeruption. The development of anterior tooth relationships, including the amount of vertical overlap, depends on skeletal form and on tongue and lip activity. Deep overbite may also arise in a previously normal occlusion affected by anterior tooth migration and overeruption.

If trauma supervenes, it may be characterized by injury both to soft tissues and teeth: gingival abrasion and recession with attrition of root surfaces, either palatally in the upper anterior segment, or labially in the lower anterior segment. Food impaction is a frequent source of acute pain and swelling, and may contribute to the development of periodontitis with recurrent periodontal abscesses. The likelihood of gingival trauma occurring is increased by loss of posterior support and by clenching or grinding habits.

Treatment

Successful treatment is dependent not only on the relief of trauma and control of infection but also on the establishment of stable centric contacts.

The first treatment option in young patients with traumatic overbite should be orthodontic therapy, perhaps involving intrusion of anterior teeth or extrusion of posterior teeth, uprighting of tilted incisors and reduction of overjet. Severe cases may require orthognathic surgery.

Many adults with deep overbite have excellent occlusal function without trauma and should not normally be offered treatment prophylactically. If trauma has occurred, it may be relieved by grinding the incisal edges of impinging incisors or, where this is impracticable, by fitting a posterior onlay appliance to increase the vertical dimension of occlusion, making sure that appropriate steps are taken to prevent further incisor extrusion. Very occasionally, if there is an associated posterior centric interference with an anterior adaptive path of closure, occlusal adjustment may be attempted to reposition the mandible distally.

Whatever methods are used to eliminate or control the impinging overbite, among those described above, it is *imperative* that steps are also taken to prevent incisor overeruption. The problem of further extrusion is usually limited to the lower incisors since the upper incisors are prevented from overerup tion by the muscle tone of the lower lip, except where there is a very high lip line as in some Angle Class II division 2 malocclusions. Stability of the lower incisors may be achieved by fitting, as a night-guard, an upper acrylic splint with an anterior bite plane to occlude against lower incisors. If there are missing teeth, the metal base of an upper partial denture can be designed to occlude against the lower incisors or else a close fitting lingual plate connector of a lower partial denture may prevent incisor overeruption. Another means of stabilizing shortened lower incisors involves the use of a resin-retained splint extending distally in the lower arch until teeth with stable centric contacts are included.

Conclusion

Deep traumatic overbite is a multidisciplinary problem. It may occur in patients with good plaque control and good gingival conditions as well as in patients with poor plaque control and gingivitis. Healthy gingivae, however, are more resistant to mechanical stress and food impaction than diseased gingivae, and so the maintenance of good oral hygiene and good periodontal conditions may help to reduce the incidence of this form of occlusal trauma.

Recall maintenance

Since the bacteria causing periodontal disease belong to the indigenous flora, they will persist in the mouth even when complete periodontal health has been established. If an adequate level of plaque control is not maintained, periodontal disease will recur.

Several factors can lead to a breakdown in plaque control: they include a failure of motivation, failure to remember oral hygiene instructions, and the gradual accumulation of calculus deposits, which provide retention sites for plaque. A programme of maintenance care, therefore, should incorporate dental health education, reinstruction, scaling and polishing, including subgingival scaling if appropriate. Recall maintenance is now sometimes referred to as 'supportive periodontal therapy'.

Objectives of maintenance care

The recall programme should be designed to maintain the degree of periodontal health which was achieved during the treatment phase. The objectives of the maintenance phase will, therefore, depend on the success of the treatment phase.

Maintenance care is necessary for all patients: those who have been rendered relatively free of periodontal disease; and those in whom the inflammatory process has been 'contained' rather than eradicated. The maintenance regimen chosen will depend on the amount of disease originally present, the extent to which it has been eliminated by treatment, the amount of time and effort previously invested in treatment, and the clinician's subjective assessment of the risk of recurrence.

Two approaches to recall maintenance will now be described: for patients with optimum periodontal health; and for patients with inadequate plaque control and a significant amount of persisting disease.

Patients with healthy periodontal tissue

Frequency of recall visits

Where optimum periodontal health has been achieved, the recall intervals should be tailored to suit individual needs. Patients who have been subjected to periodontal surgery and who are using chlorhexidine mouthwash during the immediate postoperative period should be re-examined 3 or 4 weeks after stopping the mouthwash to make sure that their plaque control methods are adequate to cope with the altered gingival architecture. During the next few months, as healing proceeds, recall intervals should be gradually increased, according to the patient's ability to sustain motivation and the rapidity with which calculus accumulates. In the long term, it is rarely practicable to provide recall prophylaxis at less than 3-month intervals and probably unwise to allow the interval to exceed one year. If, at any visit, there is evidence of periodontal breakdown, the recall frequency should be increased.

Practical recall procedures

Assuming that tooth surface débridement has been carried out adequately during the treatment phase, the critical factor determining the long-term success of periodontal therapy is the standard of self-performed plaque control practised by the patient on a daily basis. Recall visits are a means of encouraging the patient to evaluate and, if necessary, adjust tooth-cleaning techniques. Furthermore, at sites of recurrent periodontitis, subgingival instrumentation can be provided while the lesion is at an early stage and before deep-seated disease becomes re-established.

During the treatment phase, when the tissue is loose and oedematous and subgingival calculus is present, curettes with relatively large blades are used. During the maintenance phase, however, when subgingival calculus is minimal and the tissues are less easily retracted, use of these same instruments is neither necessary nor indeed practicable. Finer instruments are required, and should be employed as gently as possible.

When the maintenance programme and the patient's attention to oral hygiene are sufficient to maintain a physiological gingival sulcus, attachment loss will not occur and there is little point, therefore, in monitoring attachment levels; attachment loss is difficult and time-consuming to measure since it involves identification of the amelocemental junction as well as the base of the pocket. A pocket depth record should, nevertheless, be kept of any sites which bleed on probing. A note should also be made if any of these sites is affected by gingival recession. Then, at later recall visits, if the frequency or depth of bleeding pockets has increased, or gingival recession has occurred without an equivalent reduction in probing depth, this will be evidence that the maintenance programme is failing not only to maintain healthy conditions but also to contain recurrent disease. In these circumstances, treatment of a more intensive nature than can be provided within the recall programme, is required.

The following protocol is suggested for recall visits.

1. Initial discussion with the patient to identify new or recurrent oral problems.
2. Identification of sites of supragingival plaque accumulation and gingivitis. Reinforcement of plaque control procedures.
3. Identification and removal of supragingival calculus.
4. Identification of pathological pockets. Subgingival scaling and root planing as necessary.
5. Assessment of restorations, removal of overhangs, etc.
6. Assessment of mobility levels and of teeth subject to migration. Occlusal treatment, if necessary.
7. Polishing all accessible surfaces.
8. Treatment of sensitive teeth.
9. Decision on timing of next recall appointment.

Patients with persisting disease

Maintenance care for patients with many residual pathological pockets may simply become an extension of the treatment phase, with repeated scaling and reinforced oral hygiene instruction to maintain the level of improvement achieved during treatment or, more realistically, to retard further deterioration. A major problem is how to administer the maintenance care to greatest effect in one visit (if possible) when multiple deep pockets are present and oral hygiene is unsatisfactory.

Removal of supragingival calculus can be carried out quickly and atraumatically and should facilitate daily personal oral hygiene. In addition, the patient's impression of oral cleanliness may motivate him to a better standard of home care.

If instrumentation has been carried out adequately in the treatment phase, leaving a hard, smooth root surface, fresh subgingival deposits should be comparatively easy to remove without significant removal of root substance. On the other hand, repeated instrumentation may result in accidental destruction of fibre attachment.

Although subgingival instrumentation cannot be fully effective at sites of persistent plaque accumulation, it may produce a temporary remission. Experiments have shown that several weeks may elapse before the main periodontal pathogens are re-established in the proportions observed prior to débridement. There is, however, no satisfactory evidence that subgingival débridement, performed at regular intervals, will reduce the rate of attachment loss specifically at pockets which repeatedly become repopulated by bacteria.

Since the benefits of repeated subgingival débridement for patients with inadequate oral hygiene are, at best, uncertain, encouragement to perform better oral hygiene should receive the highest priority. Eventually, this may lead to a change in behaviour and improved oral hygiene, thereby creating suitable conditions for successful definitive instrumentation, with or without surgical access. Then, with the mouth in a more stable, healthy condition, recall maintenance will become more rational and more effective.

Acute inflammatory conditions

Acute necrotizing ulcerative gingivitis (ANUG)

Clinical features

ANUG produces characteristic signs and symptoms, which usually make diagnosis relatively easy (Fig. 20.1(a)). It is a disease of sudden onset.

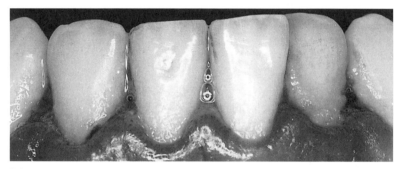

(a)

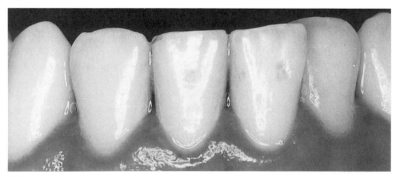

(b)

Fig. 20.1 ANUG: (a) before treatment; plaque, gingivitis and papillary ulceration are evident; (b) one month after treatment, gingivae appear normal.

Physical signs. Initially, the gingivae become red and shiny and bleed easily. The ulcers form first on interdental papillae. With increasing severity, they spread to involve the marginal gingivae and, ultimately, in some untreated cases, the attached gingivae. The ulcers are extremely painful. They are ragged in outline and are covered with a so-called 'pseudomembranous' slough which consists of infected necrotic tissue and can be wiped off the surface of the ulcer, leaving a raw, bleeding, painful area. The condition is very destructive and may leave the interdental papillae affected by 'punched-out' crater-like depressions. If inadequately treated, this characteristic deformity may persist.

There is usually a degree of submental or submandibular lymphadenitis. In the more severe cases, there may be some cervical lymphadenitis, but systemic disturbance, if any, is mild.

Although ANUG-affected sites are associated with greater attachment loss than unaffected sites in the same mouth, it has not been determined whether ANUG may result in attachment loss or simply has a predilection for sites of pre-existing attachment loss and deeper pockets. Often, 'necrotizing ulcerative periodontitis', or a similar expression, is used to describe those cases which are associated with attachment loss.

Symptoms. Pain and extreme tenderness, even to gentle probing, are common and are important diagnostic signs in incipient ANUG, which may otherwise resemble chronic gingivitis. In most cases of ANUG there is a distinctive 'foetor oris'. The patient may also complain of an unpleasant or metallic taste.

Occurrence

The incidence of the disease is roughly equal in males and females. In developed countries, the great majority of patients with ANUG are between the ages of 18 and 30 years. It is rare in young children, the middle-aged and elderly. Recurrent episodes of ANUG are common unless adequate treatment is provided. In deprived regions of Africa, where malnutrition and infectious diseases are common, ANUG may affect young children, and may spread to involve the facial tissues. This condition is referred to as 'cancrum oris' or 'noma'.

Aetiology

The aetiology of ANUG is not entirely understood. It is considered to be a fuso-spirochaetal infection of gingival tissue which, for reasons unknown, has lowered resistance to infection. The following appear to be the most significant aetiological factors.

Inadequate oral hygiene. The majority of ANUG cases occur in neglected mouths with inadequate plaque control. In a very few cases, however, areas of localized plaque retention may be present in an otherwise clean mouth. In such cases, the condition may be restricted to these zones. This would explain the occasional observation of ANUG around partially erupted lower wisdom teeth and imbricated incisors.

Fuso-spirochaetal complex. When the slough is wiped from the surface of the ulcers, and is examined microscopically, an overgrowth of various microorganisms is observed, among which spirochaetes and fusiform bacilli are prominent. The spirochaetes have not been fully characterized, but a variety of different organisms are thought to contribute to the fusiform component, including *Fusobacterium nucleatum, Selenomonas* species, *Prevotella intermedia* and *Porphyromonas gingivalis.* Spirochaetes may even be seen invading the superficial layers of inflamed gingiva beneath the pseudomembrane. The consistent observation that these organisms are present in the slough led to the early supposition that they were the causative agents and that ANUG was contagious. However, attempts to reproduce the disease in healthy volunteers by transfer of fuso-spirochaetal organisms have failed. Spirochaetes and fusiforms belong to the indigenous flora and are present in mature plaque, but the reason for their apparent overgrowth in ANUG is not clear.

Smoking. ANUG occurs predominantly in smokers, perhaps because of reduced tissue resistance due to the constrictive effects of smoking on the gingival microcirculation, or because of functional defects in peripheral blood polymorphonuclear leucocytes, caused by tobacco metabolites.

Mental stress. Although ANUG is thought sometimes to be precipitated by stress, the mechanism by which stress leads to disease is not known. Stress may cause altered peripheral blood flow and immune function, as well as increased smoking and decreased oral hygiene.

Underlying systemic disease. When host resistance is impaired, the likelihood of severe gingival and periodontal disease is increased. Thus, any patient, not responding as well as expected to local or systemic treatment for ANUG, should be investigated further. Occasionally, gingival ulceration with a fibrinous pseudomembrane may be the earliest sign of acute leukaemia, and individuals infected with human immunodeficiency virus (HIV), even those who have not developed AIDS, may be predisposed to ANUG. HIV-seropositive subjects, furthermore, are at risk from a severe necrotizing periodontitis (see below) which may manifest as ANUG in its early stages.

Treatment

The treatment of ANUG varies with the severity of the condition. In all cases, local treatment is essential and, at least in the more severe cases, systemic antimicrobial treatment is also indicated.

Local treatment. The affected area should be thoroughly débrided over a period of a few visits, at each visit carrying out as much treatment as the discomfort felt by the patient will allow. Initially, an ultrasonic scaler should be used to minimize discomfort and for the cleansing action of its spray. Gradually, the area should be cleaned more thoroughly until the lesions resolve.

In severe cases it may be possible only to remove loose debris with cotton wool pellets soaked in 3% hydrogen peroxide: the effervescence of the solution physically cleanses the area and the nascent oxygen released may be effective against anaerobic bacteria.

Oral hygiene instruction. Depending on the severity of the pain, it may be necessary to recommend a soft toothbrush. Interdental cleaning is essential to achieve a good result and should be commenced as soon as discomfort allows.

Mouthwashes. An oxidizing mouthwash such as sodium perborate (Bocasan) may be helpful in dislodging the slough and may have a direct antimicrobial effect on the anaerobic bacteria which inhabit the ulcer. Prolonged use should be avoided because of the risk of borate poisoning.

Chlorhexidine mouthwash should be prescribed to support the patient's plaque control efforts, but it will have no direct action on the infected gingivae since it does not penetrate the slough and is inactivated by necrotic tissue.

Systemic treatment. If adequate débridement is carried out, systemic treatment should be unnecessary. However, rapid resolution is desirable because of the destructive nature of the disease, and there would seem to be little point in withholding systemic antimicrobial therapy. Metronidazole is the drug of choice and is usually administered in 200-mg doses, three times daily for three days. Penicillin is a suitable alternative.

The use of drugs in the treatment of ANUG, to the exclusion of simultaneous local débridement, must be deplored since it leads, in many cases, to recurrent episodes of the disease with periods of remission (during drug therapy) which are so short as to create a false impression of a chronic condition.

Follow-up care. The treatment of ANUG is not complete until a gingival architecture has been established which will allow adequate home care. Once the ulcers have healed, careful evaluation of the periodontal tissues should establish the likelihood of achieving a normal gingival architecture. Where soft-tissue craters are comparatively shallow and interdental oral hygiene is not seriously compromised, the chances of papillary regeneration are excellent (see Fig. 20.1(b)). This process, however, may take many weeks and, since it will be inhibited by interdental plaque, close patient supervision is necessary. Surgical intervention may be required for deep soft-tissue craters and a gingivectomy or flap procedure should be chosen in accordance with the principles expressed in Chapter 11, with the objective of achieving a physiological gingival sulcus and a gingival contour which will facilitate home care.

Periodontal diseases associated with HIV

HIV-seropositive individuals are at greater risk from various oral lesions and these become more prevalent as the CD4 lymphocyte count decreases. These lesions include:

> *Oral lesions associated with HIV*
> * Acute pseudomembranous candidiasis
> * Herpes simplex infection
> * Herpes zoster infection
> * Hairy leucoplakia
> * Kaposi's sarcoma
> * Recurrent oral ulceration
> * Gingival erythema
> * ANUG/P

Gingival erythema and ANUG/P (acute necrotizing ulcerative gingivitis/periodontitis) are described briefly below. Neither of these lesions is a specific manifestation of HIV infection: they may occur both in HIV-negative immunocompromised subjects and in healthy adults.

Gingival erythema

A diffuse or punctate erythema may affect the attached gingiva and is thought to be caused by infection with *Candida albicans*. It is unresponsive to dental plaque control and requires antifungal therapy.

ANUG/P

ANUG occurs more frequently in HIV-positive subjects and is more likely to involve the supporting tissues. Furthermore, ANUP may progress rapidly with denudation and sequestration of alveolar bone. Pain and spontaneous bleeding are common. This may be regarded as a half-way stage between ANUG and cancrum oris. Indeed, if inadequately treated, ANUP may progress beyond the mucogingival junction to cause massive destruction of oral soft-tissues and underlying bone, and may be life-threatening.

The treatment of ANUP is based on the treatment of ANUG. Necrotic tissue, including loose bone sequestra, should be removed under local anaesthesia. Povidone-iodine may be preferred to hydrogen peroxide for professional débridement of the lesions, since it provides better pain relief, and chlorhexidine mouthwash is invaluable for plaque control. Local treatment should be supported by a 3–7-day course of metronidazole Broad-spectrum antibiotics may predispose to fungal infection and should be avoided.

The prevalence and severity of *chronic* gingivitis and *chronic* periodontitis in HIV-positive individuals does not appear to be substantially greater than in the general population. Indeed, gingival erythema and the ulcerative periodontal lesions described above are not, themselves, particularly common. Their presence in patients whose HIV status is unknown should alert the clinician to the possibility of other oral lesions which may suggest a diagnosis of HIV-infection.

Acute herpetic stomatitis

Acute herpetic stomatitis is a systemic infection with the herpes simplex virus (type 1, usually) which is manifest by widespread intraoral vesicles and ulceration. It is not a form of plaque-associated periodontal disease but is considered here because the lesions may affect the gingiva predominantly and cause diagnostic confusion with ANUG.

Aetiology

Acute herpetic stomatitis is essentially a disease of early childhood, when the symptoms are usually mild and often dismissed as 'teething'. However, as a result of improved living conditions, there is a reduced incidence in childhood and an increasing number of cases are diagnosed in adulthood, when the symptoms tend to be more severe. The virus is transmitted by contact with infected saliva. Virtually all adults have antibodies to this virus, indicating that they have suffered a primary infection at some time, albeit a mild one.

Clinical features

In a severe case, the onset is sudden, with high fever, cervical lymphadenopathy and pain in the mouth and throat. The gingivae may become acutely inflamed, oedematous, and tender. Intra-epithelial vesicles form within 24 hours, usually on the tongue, buccal mucosa, palate and gingivae. The vesicles rupture early, giving numerous small round or irregular superficial ulcers which may coalesce. The ulcers have a greyish-yellow base and a distinct red halo. Sometimes the gingiva may remain red and painful without evidence of ulceration. Pain may interfere with eating, drinking and swallowing. Usually the diagnosis can be made on clinical grounds alone. Various laboratory tests are available for atypical cases.

A number of features of acute herpetic stomatitis distinguish it from ANUG. Systemic symptoms are more common and more severe; ulcers may affect not only the marginal gingiva, but also the attached gingiva and other parts of the oral mucosa; the gingival lesions are not necrotic and heal without residual deformity. Unlike ANUG, acute herpetic stomatitis is a self-limiting condition which resolves in 1 or 2 weeks.

About 30% of individuals suffer recurrent infections later in life. These usually take the form of 'cold sores' on the lips (herpes labialis) but may present intraorally without significant systemic upset as a cluster of small, shallow ulcers with red irregular margins, typically on the palate or gingiva.

Treatment

Treatment of acute herpetic stomatitis is supportive and includes a soft diet with adequate fluid intake. Bed rest and analgesics may also be necessary. Oral ulceration is managed with chlorhexidine mouthwash which will reduce secondary bacterial infection and maintain dental plaque control. The antiviral agent, acyclovir, is reserved mainly for immunocompromised patients, when it may be given orally or intravenously. To be effective in non-immunocompromised patients, oral acyclovir must be administered early in the course of the disease.

The periodontal abscess

In this chapter, the term 'periodontal abscess' refers to an infection where the gingival sulcus or periodontal pocket is the point of entry of the causative organisms or their toxic products.

The periodontal abscess is an acute suppurative inflammatory lesion in which bacteria from the sulcus or pocket activate overwhelming tissue destructive processes within the gingivae or deeper periodontal tissues. Extensive tissue invasion by subgingival bacteria has not been demonstrated, although bacteria can usually be cultured from pus samples. A wide variety of organisms may be isolated in a pure or mixed infection.

Most periodontal abscesses arise as an acute exacerbation of chronic periodontitis following trauma to the epithelial lining of the pocket, and/or interruption to the flow of inflammatory exudate due to obstruction of the pocket orifice. Trauma may be caused by toothbrush bristles, food impaction, orthodontic or occlusal forces and dental procedures including scaling.

Diagnosis

The periodontal abscess has a sudden onset. Pain is present on biting and on percussion and may be continuous. There is

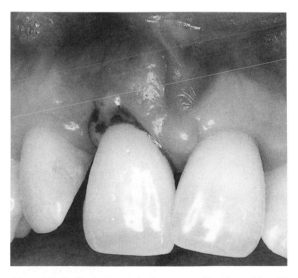

Fig. 20.2 Periodontal abscess affecting 11 with drainage of pus through the pocket orifice.

usually swelling and tenderness of the overlying gingiva (Fig. 20.2). Periodontal abscesses usually drain along the root surface to the pocket orifice although, in the case of deep pockets, they may drain through the alveolar process to produce a sinus opening in the attached gingiva. Because drainage usually occurs readily, the infection tends to remain localized. Extraoral swelling is uncommon.

There are no special radiographic features, although abscesses are commonly associated with deep pockets and, therefore, with advanced marginal bone loss.

The periodontal abscess must be differentiated from an abscess of pulpal origin. The dental abscess is associated with a non-vital pulp and usually presents as a periapical radiolucent lesion. Drainage tends to occur through alveolar mucosa or attached gingiva rather than the gingival sulcus. Dental abscesses may also occur on the lateral aspect of the root or in the furcation region if associated with lateral or accessory canals. This may lead to considerable diagnostic difficulty (see Chapter 14).

Treatment

The prognosis is poor if bone destruction is well advanced when extraction may be the treatment of choice. Otherwise, rigorous treatment must be provided.

Drainage can usually be encouraged by dilating the pocket with a periodontal probe or flat plastic instrument, but fluctuant mucosal swellings should be incised. Gentle subgingival scaling should be carried out to remove calculus and foreign objects, if present. The patient should be advised to use hot saline mouthwashes at home, and these measures together will usually relieve the symptoms quickly, although analgesics may be necessary. Systemic antimicrobial therapy, while not usually necessary, should, nevertheless, be considered so that all possible steps are taken to limit the permanent destruction of fibre attachment and improve the prognosis. Penicillin or metronidazole are the drugs of choice, and will certainly be required for cellulitis or pyrexia. The patient should return 2 days later to have local treatment repeated. Overenthusiastic instrumentation should be avoided since it may result in penetration of the 'soft' base of the pocket and destruction of viable tissue.

As the symptoms resolve, oral hygiene instruction and superficial scaling should continue until sufficient time has elapsed for healing of the abscess site – about 2 months. Successful treatment is recognized by a considerable reduction in probing depth. A pathological pocket, albeit with a reduced depth, may still exist and should be subjected to definitive treatment according to the principles expressed in Chapter 8. This may involve subgingival scaling and root planing, or surgical intervention.

Sometimes the acute symptoms disappear but a chronic draining lesion remains. This may signify a continuing, rapid, destructive process and may be a sign of bad prognosis. To arrest the destructive process in these cases, early surgical intervention is indicated following satisfactory completion of hygiene therapy and preparation of a definitive treatment plan.

Where the infection is severe or the patient immunocompromised, pus may be collected from a discharging sinus or, by needle aspiration, from a fluctuant swelling. Then, if the lesion fails to respond to treatment, and a change of antibiotic has to be considered, culture and sensitivity test results will be available.

Periodontal aspects of restorative dentistry

Restorations and prostheses should be designed not only to minimize plaque accumulation in the proximity of the marginal periodontal tissues but also to avoid physical injury to the gingiva and periodontal ligament. This chapter is devoted to a consideration of gingival margin–restoration relationships, to discussion of the support potential of the reduced periodontium, and to a brief consideration of dental implants.

Periodontal care of teeth with subgingival restorations

Once caries has been excavated and undermined enamel removed, cavity margins often extend subgingivally. There is great individual variation in periodontal tissue response to subgingival restorations. Their effects will depend to a large extent on the care taken to achieve an accurately fitting restoration, free from surface imperfections as far as possible. However, even a perfectly formed restoration will likely retain some plaque subgingivally at the tooth–restoration interface, cause some degree of gingivitis and may initiate a destructive periodontal lesion.

This problem may be addressed by carrying out a surgical procedure designed to locate the gingival margin in a more apical position, thereby exposing the whole restoration. The complexity of such a procedure depends on the distance between the bone margin and the restoration, since a space of 3–4 mm is required to accommodate a normal height of gingival tissue. Therefore, a restoration margin which lies within this 3–4 mm zone cannot be exposed permanently by excision or apical positioning of gingival tissue, unless some underlying bone is also removed. Such a step is not usually justifiable since many gingival pockets, even without treatment, will not progress to destructive periodontitis. Of course, *soft tissue* surgery may still be worthwhile if only to gain temporary exposure of the restoration to correct a faulty margin or construct a better fitting replacement.

The harmful effects of a subgingival restoration can, to some extent, be mitigated by the daily use of dental floss interproximally within the pocket and employment of the Bass technique of intrasulcular brushing (see Fig. 9.1) for buccal and lingual surfaces.

Crown margins

The case for a *supragingival* margin in the restoration of carious teeth applies even more to elective crown preparation. If a retentive preparation is created supragingivally, impression procedures, temporary crown provision and final cementation will all be greatly simplified. In addition, the marginal seal may be inspected without difficulty, a factor of special importance for bridge retainers which may undergo cementation failure while remaining *in situ*, attached to other parts of the bridge.

Whenever possible, therefore, all crown restorations should be designed with a supragingival margin, with the possible exception of upper anterior and premolar crowns, where it may be necessary for aesthetic reasons, to conceal the labial margin just within the gingival sulcus (Fig. 21.1). Provided the preparation extends no more than 0.5 mm apical to the gingival crest (i.e. no deeper than the base of the histological sulcus), little harm will result, although a mild gingivitis is virtually inevitable.

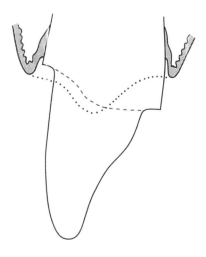

Fig. 21.1 Sagittal section through an anterior jacket crown preparation. The buccal finishing line is located within the gingival sulcus. The lingual finishing line is located in a supragingival position. Outside the plane of section, the dotted line represents the outline of the interdental gingival margin and the broken line represents the interdental cervical margin of the crown preparation.

On the other hand, deliberate subgingival extension beyond the base of the sulcus with disruption of the epithelial attachment is to be condemned. This will lead to subgingival plaque accumulation and gingivitis, possibly to be followed by periodontitis and/or gingival recession. Indeed, it is well established that deeply placed subgingival margins on labial tooth surfaces may promote gingival recession and so defeat the original purpose of aesthetic restoration.

Although crown construction is always easier when carried out wholly on the visible tooth surface, the operative work is unlikely to be seriously compromised by a subgingival extension of up to 0.5 mm. The result should be an accurately fitting crown with a highly polished or glazed surface located at the front of the mouth, where the patient has optimum access to clean the crown margin with an intrasulcular technique such as the Bass method. Subgingival placement of anterior jacket crown margins should not, however, extend to the proximal or palatal aspects, where a supragingival finishing line is desirable for minimal interference with gingival health (Fig. 21.1).

Surgical crown lengthening

When the remaining clinical crown is too short to achieve a retentive preparation and the occlusion is such that an adequate core cannot be built up, surgical crown lengthening should be considered. As described above, it will be necessary to allow for normal gingival dimensions or 'biologic width' to be established during healing. Thus, a bone to gingival margin distance of approximately 3 mm on facial and lingual surfaces, and 4 mm on proximal surfaces must be allowed for.

Except where gingival enlargement or periodontal pockets of sufficient depth are already present, the marginal bone height must be reduced (usually by 2 or 3 mm), following flap reflection. Diamond stones should be used with copious irrigation to reduce and thin the marginal bone, with the final edge of bone being removed with hand instruments in order to avoid bur marks on the root surface. The newly exposed root surface should be curetted to remove remnants of periodontal ligament which might encourage regeneration of bone.

The gingival margin can be positioned more apically either by excision of soft tissue or, where gingivectomy would leave an inadequate width of attached gingiva, by an apically repositioned flap procedure.

When periodontal surgery has been carried out, definitive anterior crown preparation should ideally be delayed for at least

20 weeks in order to allow the position of the gingival crest to stabilize fully.

Support potential of the reduced periodontium

In this section 'reduced periodontium' refers to a situation where there is a marked reduction in number of teeth or severe attachment loss, thereby reducing the periodontal support available for a partial prosthesis.

Fixed or removable?

In general, a fixed bridge is preferable to a removable partial denture. It is less obtrusive, causes less enhancement of plaque accumulation and is, therefore, less likely to promote periodontal disease. On the other hand, more clinical and technical expertise is required, and the cost implications are greater.

There was a tendency in the past to reserve bridgework for short spans where the abutment teeth had good periodontal support, and to construct removable partial dentures for patients whose abutment teeth were few in number or poorly supported. However, the shortcomings of partial dentures are even more obvious in cases of reduced periodontal support. Where edentulous free-end saddle areas or other long spans exist, flexure or tilting of the denture base is likely. This may result in gingival and mucosal trauma. Soft-tissue trauma may also result from denture movement as teeth, already mobile, are rocked by denture components such as clasp arms and connectors. In theory, this should not occur if proper reciprocation is employed. In practice, a period of periodontal 'adaptation' often follows the insertion of a new partial denture, at the end of which abutment teeth may be so mobile that retention and support are compromised, and gingival trauma arises as a result of movement of the denture base in function. This problem may be overcome by provision of fixed bridgework of cross-arch design.

Advantages of bridgework

Although the above mentioned drawbacks of partial dentures are well recognized and fully acknowledged, prosthodontists have felt constrained by 'Ante's law' from providing fixed bridgework in cases of reduced periodontal support. Ante proposed that, in a fixed bridge the root surface area of the abutment teeth should be equal to or greater than the root surface area of the teeth to be replaced by pontics. While this may be considered safe advice, there is no doubt that such a rigid formula places considerable constraints on abutment selection. At the other extreme, it has been shown that, provided healthy periodontal conditions are achieved and maintained, satisfactory function can be restored with bridges which rely for their support on as little as 16% of the presumed root surface area of the teeth being replaced by pontics. Thus, bridgework is possible and, indeed, preferable even for patients with reduced periodontal support. This is especially so when there is significant tooth mobility, since the greater rigidity of the fixed reconstruction provides a more favourable distribution of masticatory function to the remaining periodontium.

Notwithstanding the clinical and technical difficulties of fixed bridgework in general, the *reduced* periodontium may afford certain advantages to the clinician and technician. Increased clinical crown length should allow preparation of abutments with excellent retention form and, if aesthetics allow, supragingival margins. Moreover, increased vertical space will be available (owing to alveolar bone loss) to construct components of sufficient dimension to resist the deformation which can lead to fracture of metal, porcelain or cement lute. Finally, it should be noted that mechanoreceptors within the periodontal ligament restrict, by feedback, the amount of force generated by the muscles of mastication, and thereby, limit the load on the bridge.

Periodontal prognosis

It is, of course, essential that periodontal disease is treated successfully before a complex and costly fixed prosthesis is provided. If periodontal health cannot be achieved and advanced periodontitis persists, the prognosis for the dentition will be poor, regardless of the method chosen for tooth replacement. Then economic factors will often dictate provision of a removable prosthesis. When the prognosis is particularly poor, this should be regarded as a transitional denture, that is, a partial denture which is provided as part of a planned transition to a complete denture.

Dental implants

Earlier subperiosteal and blade-type endosteal implants have largely been superseded by parallel-sided screw and cylinder ('root form') designs which may be used for fixed single-tooth and bridge restorations, and in conjunction with removable overdenture-type prostheses. Some of these designs have been shown to achieve osseointegration or 'functional ankylosis' by means of the biocompatibility of specially prepared titanium or hydroxyapatite surfaces. Very few designs have undergone proper scientific evaluation or long-term study.

Attachment apparatus

In contrast to the ligamentous attachment of the natural tooth, osseointegration involves the complete absence of any kind of soft tissue interface between implant and bone. On the other hand, the mucosal interface with the implant, under favourable conditions, may simulate the attachment mechanisms of a natural tooth. Thus, a junctional epithelium is attached to the implant pillar by a basal lamina and hemidesmosomes. This collar of epithelium is approximately 2 mm in height and is derived from the peri-implant mucosa. Between the junctional epithelium and the bone crest, a connective tissue 'attachment' zone of approximately 1 mm is present. However, in contrast to the dentogingival attachment, collagen fibre bundles adjacent to implant surfaces usually run parallel to, rather than perpendicular to the implant surface, or are circular in orientation.

Where the implant lies in mobile, non-keratinized mucosa, the connective tissue collar may be less stable and less likely to support an epithelial attachment or to resist downgrowth of epithelium and pocket formation. The epithelial attachment serves as a barrier to bacterial penetration and, in its absence, infection and implant failure may ensue.

Although rough titanium or hydroxyapatite implant surfaces will promote osseointegration and suprabony fibre 'attachment' or adhesion, polished titanium is easier to maintain plaque-free where the implant penetrates the mucosa. Scaling, if necessary, should be carried out using specially designed plastic scalers to avoid scratching the transmucosal implant surface. There is now some evidence that the hydroxyapatite coating used in some implant systems may disintegrate after a number of years and lead to implant failure.

Peri-implant probing

The condition of the peri-implant tissue should be monitored in a manner similar to periodontal tissue. This will include probing, but a lighter force should be used since healthy peri-implant soft tissues offer less resistance to probing. A probing depth of approximately 3 mm is normal.

Peri-implant disease

Apart from early postoperative wound infection, two forms of peri-implant disease can be recognized: plaque-induced disease, and bone loss due to overloading. These may arise separately or in combination.

Plaque-induced disease may take two forms, *peri-implant mucositis*, which is reversible, and *peri-implantitis* which is not. These conditions are equivalent to the gingivitis and periodontitis which affect natural teeth. Thus, plaque accumulation causes peri-implant mucositis, and if not treated, the chronic infection may extend subgingivally causing peri-implantitis. This may be untreatable if the infection is allowed to reach the lumen of hollow implants. Ultimately loosening of the implant may occur or acute infection may supervene. The early signs of peri-implantitis are as follows:

Signs of peri-implantitis
- The peri-implant mucosa may be inflamed and swollen.
- Bleeding after gentle probing.
- Exudation and suppuration from the implant space.
- Increase in probing depth related to a fixed reference point on the implant (loss of 'attachment').
- Radiographic evidence of angular bone defects.

Early plaque-induced disease may respond to conventional periodontal treatment. If angular bone defects are present, guided tissue regeneration techniques (Chapter 12) may permit bone-fill with osseous re-integration, and prevent epithelialization of the exposed implant surface. Persistent or recurrent infection, however, with loosening of the implant, necessitates its removal to avoid excessive bone loss.

If the peri-implant soft tissue is composed of relatively mobile and non-keratinized alveolar mucosa, oral hygiene procedures may be difficult, resulting in trauma or plaque accumulation and inflammation. These mucogingival problems may occur, either when implants have been located within or adjacent to alveolar mucosa, or owing to gingival recession. The latter may result in exposure of the rough osteo-inductive implant surface causing enhanced plaque accumulation, an intractable mucosal problem and a high risk of progressive peri-implant disease. The treatment of mucogingival problems, including gingival augmentation surgery, is described in Chapter 17.

Biomechanical overload. Implant loosening may also result from premature loading before osseointegration has occurred, or later, from torque applied by poorly fitting superstructures or by inadequately designed occlusal schemes which ignore the need for axial loading. It is difficult to stabilize loose implants and early removal should be considered.

Periodontal screening

Screening is a procedure designed for symptomless individuals to identify those with sufficient signs of disease to justify further investigation or preventive or therapeutic intervention. Current systems of periodontal screening are based on the Community Periodontal Index of Treatment Needs (CPITN).

CPITN

The CPITN was introduced by the World Health Organization in 1982 to provide data on treatment needs so that health authorities could develop appropriate preventive and treatment services for large communities.

Three indicators of periodontal status are used: gingival bleeding, calculus and periodontal pockets. Examination is carried out using a specially designed probe with a colour band 3.5–5.5 mm from the end, and with a ball tip for calculus detection (Fig. AI.1). The dentition is divided into sextants, comprising the two anterior and four posterior segments. The entire circumference of each tooth is probed and, using the scoring criteria described in Table AI.1, a score is given to each sextant according to the worst finding in that sextant. The scores are recorded on a simple box chart (Fig. AI.2). A sextant containing only one tooth is recorded as missing (x) and the tooth is examined and scored along with those in the adjacent sextant.

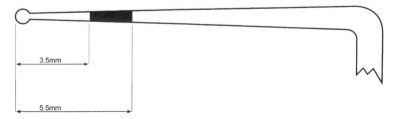

Fig. AI.1 The WHO periodontal probe for CPITN scoring.

Table AI.1 *Scoring criteria for CPITN*

CPITN code	Probing depth	Calculus or defective margin	Bleeding on probing
0	Colour band visible	No	No
1	Colour band visible	No	Yes
2	Colour band visible	Yes	–
3	Colour band partially visible	–	–
4	Colour band not visible	–	–

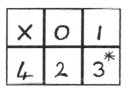

Fig. AI.2 Box chart for recording the CPITN (see text for explanation of specimen scores).

Treatment needs are based on the CPITN scores (codes) as follows:

Code 0   no treatment
Code 1   improved oral hygiene
Codes 2 + 3   improved oral hygiene and scaling and/or adjustment of restorations
Code 4   complex treatment, perhaps including surgery

Unfortunately CPITN data are insufficiently precise upon which to base a calculation of workforce requirements, time, cost and specific therapy for large population groups. It has never, therefore, been able to fulfil its intended purpose, but has, instead, been extensively used as an epidemiological tool to estimate the prevalence, severity and extent of periodontal disease. This, too, has attracted much criticism since the CPITN does not include the cumulative manifestations of periodontal destruction, such as attachment loss, gingival recession and loss of alveolar bone and, because of gingival recession, it provides an increasing underestimate of disease severity with increasing age.

The CPITN is still regarded as a valid screening tool in general practice for rapid identification of patients who require further investigations or treatment, and has been adapted specifically for this purpose by the British Society of Periodontology and by the American Academy of Periodontology in conjunction with the American Dental Association. Recognizing that complex treatment needs are not limited to teeth which score 4, these specialist bodies have made provision for recording other clinical abnormalities which may require treatment, such as furcation disease, hypermobility or a recession defect – an asterisk is placed next to the sextant score.

When the CPITN is used in general dental practice, the British Society of Periodontology recommends that sextants scoring 3 should receive more detailed examination *after* initial treatment; and if any sextant scores 4 or is given an asterisk, full clinical records should be obtained for all sextants together with necessary radiographs *before* treatment is planned. In these cases, specialist referral may also be appropriate.

Although the CPITN is thought to be useful as an initial screening tool in general dental practice, the index is too insensitive to detect the positive or negative outcomes of professional intervention, and is, therefore, of little value for monitoring periodontal conditions. A sextant initially scoring 3 (probing depth 3.5–5.5 mm) may no longer bleed on probing after treatment, but probing depth, and, therefore, the CPITN score, may remain the same. Alternatively, attachment loss may occur after treatment without any change in pocket depths, and, therefore, in CPITN scores of 3 or 4, if gingival recession occurs by the same amount. Thus periodontal conditions can become significantly better or substantially worse with no change in the index.

Key points
- The CPITN with or without modification can be used in general practice.
- It should be used purely for initial screening.
- Scores of 3, 4 or * indicate a need for more thorough examination and recording.
- It is unsuitable for monitoring the progress of the disease or its treatment.
- A CPITN record may be useful for medicolegal purposes.

Examination chart

Explanatory notes

Numerous methods exist for recording clinical periodontal data. The specimen chart (Fig. AII.1) illustrated overleaf combines the advantages of a pictorial system for rapid identification of particular teeth with space for numerical data. This system of charting, furthermore, places an emphasis on precise identification of diseased sites.

The chart may be used at the patient's first visit or at any subsequent visit, either during treatment or at recall. Use of this chart is particularly advised following completion of hygiene therapy, except for the simplest and most straightforward cases. Data are collected by making separate circuits of the mouth for each pathological feature. This is less time-consuming than collecting all the different types of data for each tooth in turn. The following examination procedure is suggested.

Missing teeth

Missing teeth are recorded by deleting the relevant portions of the charted dentition.

Plaque record

Using a 'highlighter' pen, the presence (highlighter mark) or absence (no mark) of cervical plaque should be recorded on six aspects of each tooth using the small boxes in the 'Pockets' row. This will allow the distribution of supragingival plaque to be readily viewed in relation to diseased sites.

Probing depths

Pocket charting is based on the identification of diseased sites at six points around each tooth. A diseased site is one which, regardless of probing depth, bleeds on probing, or looks

Fig. AII.1 Examination chart and pretreatment radiographs.

inflamed (even if bleeding does not occur). The presence of a diseased site is noted by recording its probing depth even if that amounts to no more than 1 mm. Healthy sites which look uninflamed and do not bleed on probing are denoted by placing 'dots' in the appropriate boxes, regardless of their probing depths. Six aspects of every tooth are probed: distolingual, mid-lingual, mesiolingual, distobuccal, mid-buccal and mesiobuccal. This is carried out by examining an entire arch, first the lingual surfaces, probing three aspects of each tooth, and then repeating the procedure for buccal surfaces.

Mobility scores

Each tooth should be rocked between an instrument handle and index finger in a buccolingual direction (and mesiodistal direction when no adjacent tooth is present). The amplitude of tooth movement of the crown tip from its most extreme buccal (or mesial) position to its most extreme lingual (or distal) position should be observed:

Grade 1 – visible horizontal mobility up to 1 mm
Grade 2 – visible horizontal mobility between 1 mm and 2 mm
Grade 3 – visible horizontal mobility greater than 2 mm or rotation or vertical mobility (depression).

Furcation lesions

Grade 1 – up to 3 mm horizontal attachment loss
Grade 2 – over 3 mm horizontal attachment loss but not 'through-and-through'
Grade 3 – a 'through-and-through' lesion.

The furcation score is marked on the chart according to the site of the lesion, i.e. buccal, lingual, mesial or distal.

Other clinical findings (not illustrated)

According to the needs of the clinician, additional information may be obtained and recorded: caries and overhanging restorations may be marked in different colours on the relevant tooth; unerupted teeth may be circled in one colour and non-vital teeth in another.

Gingival recession and attachment level scores would normally have little effect on the treatment plan and, therefore, are not usually recorded. Nevertheless, a separate check should be made for mucogingival problems and radiographs should be consulted if doubt exists concerning tooth support.

How the examination chart contributes to the treatment plan is illustrated in Figure AII.1.

Case history and treatment plan

A 49-year-old woman had forgone dental treatment for several years as she was terrified by the prospect of dentures and, after eventually presenting for examination, required reassurance about this before she would consent to any extractions. In spite of severe periodontal breakdown and untreated caries (see radiographs in Figure AII.1), plaque control was only slightly deficient. Ignoring the molars, a short course of treatment comprising oral hygiene instruction, scaling and root planing was provided to establish optimum plaque control and remove all detectable subgingival deposits.

One month later, a detailed clinical periodontal examination was carried out to record levels of residual periodontal disease (see chart in Figure AII.1). By this time, plaque control had reached a near perfect standard. After reference to mounted study casts, together with the clinical and radiographic findings, a treatment plan was presented to the patient and subsequently carried out:

1. Root canal therapy for non-vital 43.
2. Linked temporary crowns: 43, 44, 45 to stabilize 45 and improve occlusal function.
3. Temporary bridge construction to replace missing teeth and improve tooth stability and occlusal function: 11, 13, 14, 15 and 32, 34, 35.
4. Further non-surgical root débridement: 11, 25.
5. Open flap curettage: 13, 14, 15 with extraction of 16.
6. Open flap curettage: 43, 44, 45 with extraction of 47, 48.
7. Open flap curettage: 34, 35 with extraction of 27, 36, 37.
8. Recall maintenance and observation.
9. Wait 6 months to confirm that stable, healthy, periodontal conditions have been achieved then replace the temporary acrylic prostheses with metal-ceramic restorations, adjusting cervical preparation margins as necessary.

The result is depicted in the 3-year follow-up radiographs (Fig. AII.2).

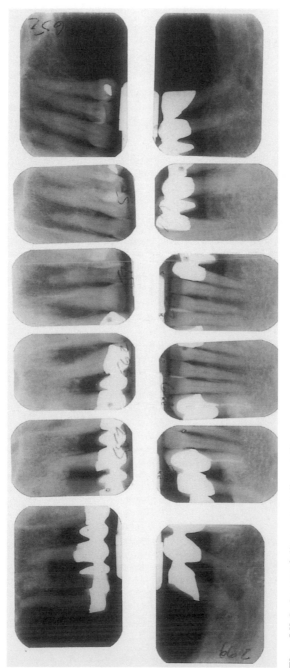

Fig. AII.2 3-year follow-up radiographs.

Further reading

Chapter 1

Schroeder, H.E. (ed.) (1997). Biological structure of the normal and diseased periodontium. *Periodontology 2000*, **13**, 1–148.

Chapter 2

Kinane, D.F. and Lindhe, J. (1997). Pathogenesis of periodontitis. In *Clinical Periodontology and Implant Dentistry* (Lindhe, J., Karring, T., Lang, N.P. eds). pp. 190–225, Copenhagen: Munksgaard.

Kornman, K.S., Page, R.C. and Tonetti, M.S. (1997). The host response to the microbial challenge in periodontitis: assembling the players. *Periodontology 2000*, **14**, 33–53.

Chapter 3

Salvi, G.E., Lawrence, H.P., Offenbacher, S. and Beck, J.D. (1997). Influence of risk factors on the pathogenesis of periodontitis. *Periodontology 2000*, **14**, 173–201.

Zambon, J.J. (1996). Periodontal diseases: microbial factors. *Annals of Periodontology, Volume 1: Proceedings of the 1996 World Workshop in Periodontics.* pp. 879–925, Chicago: American Academy of Periodontology.

Chapter 4

Gher, M.E. (1998). Changing concepts: the effects of occlusion on periodontitis. *The Dental Clinics of North America*, **42**, 285–299.

Giargia, M. and Lindhe, J. (1997). Tooth mobility and periodontal disease. *Journal of Clinical Periodontology*, **24**, 785–795.

Chapter 5

Papapanou, P.N. (1996). Periodontal diseases: epidemiology. In *Annals of Periodontology, Volume 1: Proceedings of the 1996 World Workshop in Periodontics.* pp. 1–36, Chicago: American Academy of Periodontology.

Position Paper (1996). Epidemiology of periodontal diseases. *Journal of Periodontology*, **67**, 935–945.

Chapter 6

Armitage, G.C. (1996). Periodontal diseases: diagnosis. *Annals of Periodontology,*

Volume 1: Proceedings of the 1996 World Workshop in Periodontics. pp. 37–215, Chicago: American Academy of Periodontology.

Hefti, A.F. (1997). Periodontal probing. *Critical Reviews in Oral Biology and Medicine,* **8,** 336–356.

Chapter 7

Caffesse, R.G., Mota, L.F. and Morrison, E.C. (1995). The rationale for periodontal therapy. *Periodontology 2000,* **9,** 7–13.

Van der Velden, U. and Schoo, W.H. (1997). Scientific basis for the treatment of periodontitis. In *Clinical Periodontology and Implant Dentistry* (Lindhe, J., Karring, T., Lang, N.P. eds). pp. 794–821, Copenhagen: Munksgaard.

Chapter 8

Position Paper (1997). Treatment of gingivitis and periodontitis. *Journal of Periodontology,* **68,** 1246–1253.

Chapter 9

Addy, M. and Moran, J.M. (eds) (1997). Toothpaste, mouthrinse and other topical remedies in periodontics. *Periodontology 2000,* **15,** 7–117.

Jenkins, W.M.M. (1996). The prevention and control of chronic periodontal disease. In *Prevention of Oral Disease,* 3rd edn (J.J.Murray, ed.). pp. 118–138, Oxford: Oxford University Press.

Lang, N.P., Attström, R. and Löe, H. (eds) (1998). *Proceedings of the European Workshop on Mechanical Plaque Control.* Berlin: Quintessence Books.

Chapter 10

Cobb, C.M. (1996). Non-surgical pocket therapy: mechanical. In *Annals of Periodontology: Proceedings of the 1996 World Workshop in Periodontics.* pp. 443–490, Chicago: American Academy of Periodontology.

Drisko, C.H. (1998). Root instrumentation: power-driven versus manual scalers, which one? *The Dental Clinics of North America,* 42, 229–244.

Chapter 11

Laurell, L., Gottlow, J., Zybutz, M. and Persson, R. (1998). Treatment of intrabony defects by different surgical procedures. A literature review. *Journal of Periodontology,* **69,** 303–313.

Palcanis, K.G. (1996). Surgical pocket therapy. In *Annals of Periodontology: Proceedings of the 1996 World Workshop in Periodontics.* pp. 589–617, Chicago: American Academy of Periodontology.

Chapter 12

Karring, T., Lindhe, J. and Cortellini, P. (1997). Regenerative periodontal therapy. In *Clinical Periodontology and Implant Dentistry,* 3rd edn, (Lindhe, J., Karring, T., Lang, N.P., eds). pp. 597–646, Copenhagen: Munksgaard.

Lang, N.P., Karring, T. and Lindhe, J. (eds) (1997). Session IV: Chemicals in periodontal regeneration. In *Proceedings of the 2nd European Workshop on Periodontology* (Ittingen, 1996). pp. 274–360, London: Quintessence Books.

Chapter 13

Carnevale, G., Pontoriero, R. and Hürzeler, M.B. (1995). Management of furcation involvement. *Periodontology 2000*, **9**, 69–89.
Newell, D.H. (1998). The diagnosis and treatment of molar furcation lesions. *The Dental Clinics of North America*, **42**, 301–337.

Chapter 14

Bergenholtz, G. and Hasselgren, G. (1997). Endodontics and periodontics. In *Clinical Periodontology and Implant Dentistry* (Lindhe, J., Karring, T., Lang, N.P. eds). pp. 296–325, Copenhagen: Munksgaard.
Paul, B.F. and Hutter, J.W. (1997). The endodontic–periodontal continuum revisited: new insights into etiology, diagnosis and treatment. *Journal of the American Dental Association*, **128**, 1541–1548.

Chapter 15

Albandar, J.M., Brown, M.J., Genco, R.J. and Löe, H. (1997). Clinical classification in adolescents and young adults. *Journal of Periodontology*, **68**, 545–555.
Schenkein, H.A. and Van Dyke, T.E. (1994). Early-onset periodontitis: systemic aspects of etiology and pathogenesis. *Periodontology 2000*, **6**, 7–25.

Chapter 16

Greenstein, G. and Polson, A. (1998). The role of local drug delivery in the management of periodontal diseases: a comprehensive review. *Journal of Periodontology*, **69**, 507–520.
Slots, J. and Rams, T.E. (eds) (1996). Systemic and topical antimicrobial therapy in periodontics. *Periodontology 2000*, **10**, 5–159.

Chapter 17

Wennström, J. and Pini Prato, G.P. (1997). Mucogingival therapy. In *Clinical Periodontology and Implant Dentistry* (Lindhe, J., Karring, T., Lang, N.P. eds). pp. 550–596, Copenhagen: Munksgaard.

Chapter 18

Gher, M.E. (1996). Non-surgical pocket therapy: dental occlusion. In *Annals of Periodontology, Volume 1: Proceedings of the 1996 World Workshop in Periodontics.* pp. 567–580, Chicago: American Academy of Periodontology.
Ong, M.A., Wang, H.-L. and Smith, F.N. (1998). Interrelationship between periodontics and adult orthodontics. *Journal of Clinical Periodontology*, **25**, 271–277.

Chapter 19

Echeverria, J.J., Manau, G.C. and Guerrero, A. (1996). Supportive care after active periodontal treatment. A review. *Journal of Clinical Periodontology*, **23**, 898–905.

Lang, N.P. and Tonetti, M.S. (1996). Periodontal diagnosis in treated periodontitis. Why, when and how to use clinical parameters. *Journal of Clinical Periodontology*, **23**, 240–250.

Wilson, T.G. Jr. (ed.) (1996). Supportive periodontal treatment and retreatment in periodontics. *Periodontology 2000*, **12**, 11–140.

Chapter 20

Murayama, Y., Kurihara, H., Atsushi, N. *et al.* (1994). Acute necrotizing ulcerative gingivitis: risk factors involving host defense mechanisms. *Periodontology 2000*, **6**, 116–124.

Robinson, P.G. (1997). Treatment of HIV-associated periodontal diseases. *Oral Diseases*, **3**, Supplement 1, 238–240.

Chapter 21

Cochran, D. (1996). Implant therapy I. In *Annals of Periodontology, Volume 1. Proceedings of the 1996 World Workshop in Periodontics.* pp. 707–791, Chicago: American Academy of Periodontology.

Lindhe, J. and Berglundh, T. (1998). The interface between the mucosa and the implant. *Periodontology 2000*, **17**, 47–54.

Meffert, R.M. (1996). Periodontitis vs peri-implantitis: The same disease? The same treatment? *Critical Reviews in Oral Biology and Medicine*, **7**, 278–291.

Wise, M.D. (1995). *Failure in the Restored Dentition: Management and Treatment.* London: Quintessence Books.

Appendix I

Periodontology in General Dental Practice in the United Kingdom: A First Policy Statement (1986, Revised 1994). London: British Society of Periodontology.

Proceedings of the 1994 CPITN Workshop (1994). *International Dental Journal*, **44**, no. 5, Supplement 1, 523–594.

Index